Stop and rest for a minute. Then try again, with the opposite arm raised this time. Again, record your observations.

Suggested timings are given for each activity. These are only a guide. You may like to note how long it took you to complete this activity, as it may help in planning the time needed for working through the sessions.

Time taken on activity

Time management is important. While we recognise that people learn at different speeds, this pack is designed to take 20 study hours (your tutor will also advise you). You should allocate time during each week for study.

Take some time now to identify likely periods that you can set aside for study during the week.

	Mon	Tues	Wed	Thurs	Fri	Sat	Sun
am							
pm							
eve							

At the end of the learning pack, there is a learning review to help you assess whether you have achieved the learning objectives.

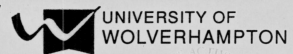
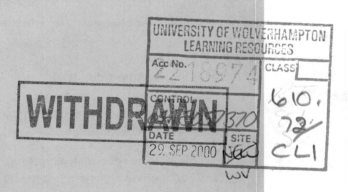

Using this workbook

The workbook is divided into 'Sessions', covering specific subjects.

In the introduction to each learning pack there is a learner profile to help you assess your current knowledge of the subjects covered in each session.

Each session has clear learning objectives. They indicate what you will be able to achieve or learn by completing that session.

Each session has a summary to remind you of the key points of the subjects covered.

Each session contains text, diagrams and learning activities that relate to the stated objectives.

It is important to complete each activity, making your own notes and writing in answers in the space provided. **Remember this is your own workbook—you are allowed to write on it**.

Now try an example activity.

ACTIVITY

This activity shows you what happens when cells work without oxygen. This really is a physical activity, so please only try it if you are fully fit.

First, raise one arm straight up in the air above your head, and let the other hand rest by your side. Clench both fists tightly, and then open out your fingers wide. Repeat this at the rate of once or twice a second. Try to keep clenching both fists at the same rate. Keep going for about five minutes, and record what you observe.

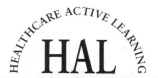

RESEARCH METHODOLOGY
in nursing and healthcare

Collette Clifford PhD MSc DANS Dip N RGN OND RNT

Reader in Health and Nursing, School of Health Studies
Faculty of Education and Health Sciences, University of Wolverhampton

Ros Carnwell MA BA RGN RHV Cert Ed

Senior Lecturer in Health Studies, School of Health Studies
Faculty of Education and Health Sciences, University of Wolverhampton

Louise Harken MSc BSc (Hons) Post Grad Dip

Demonstrator in Information Technology, School of Health Studies
Faculty of Education and Health Sciences, University of Wolverhampton

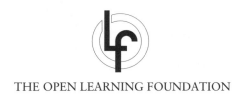

THE OPEN LEARNING FOUNDATION

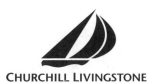

CHURCHILL LIVINGSTONE

NEW YORK EDINBURGH LONDON MADRID MELBOURNE SAN FRANCISCO AND TOKYO 1996

CHURCHILL LIVINGSTONE
Medical Division of Longman Group UK Limited

Distributed in the United States of America by Churchill
Livingstone Inc., 650 Avenue of the Americas, New York,
N.Y. 10011, and by associated companies, branches and
representatives throughout the world.

First published 1997

ISBN 0 443 05737 0

British Library of Cataloguing in Publication Data
A catalogue record for this book is available from the
British Library.

Library of Congress Cataloging in Publication Data
A catalog record for this book is available from the
Library of Congress

Produced through Longman Malaysia, PP

For The Open Learning Foundation

Director of Programmes: Leslie Mapp
Series Editor: Peter Birchenall
Programmes Manager: Kathleen Farren
Design and Production Manager: Steve Moulds

For Churchill Livingstone

Director (Nursing and Allied Health): Peter Shepherd
Project Controller: Derek Robertson
Project Manager: Valerie Burgess
Design Direction: Judith Wright
Sales Promotion Executive: Maria O' Connor

CONTENTS

OPEN LEARNING FOUNDATION TEAM MEMBERS

Writers: Collette Clifford
Reader in Health and Nursing, School of Health Studies
Faculty of Education and Health Sciences, University of Wolverhampton

Ros Carnwell
Senior Lecturer in Health Studies, School of Health Studies
Faculty of Education and Health Sciences, University of Wolverhampton

Louise Harken
Demonstrator in Information Technology, School of Health Studies
Faculty of Education and Health Sciences, University of Wolverhampton

Editor: Pip Hardy

Reviewer: Anne Lacey
Senior Lecturer in Nursing,
University of Huddersfield

Series Editor: Peter Birchenall
OLF Programme Head,
Health and Nursing,
University of Humberside

THE OPEN LEARNING FOUNDATION

Higher education has grown considerably in recent years. As well as catering for more students, universities are facing the challenge of providing for an increasingly diverse student population. Students have a wider range of backgrounds and previous educational qualifications. There are greater numbers of mature students. There is a greater need for part-time courses and continuing education and professional development programmes.

The Open Learning Foundation helps over 20 member institutions meet this growing and diverse demand – through the production of high-quality teaching and learning materials, within a strategy of creating a framework for more flexible learning. It offers member institutions the capability to increase their range of teaching options and to cover subjects in greater breadth and depth.

It does not enrol its own students. Rather, The Open Learning Foundation, by developing and promoting the greater use of open and distance learning, enables universities and others in higher education to make study more accessible and cost-effective for individual students and for business through offering more choice and more flexible courses.

Formed in 1990, the Foundation's policy objectives are to:

- improve the quality of higher education and training

- increase the quantity of higher education and training

- raise the efficiency of higher education and training delivery.

In working to meet these objectives, The Open Learning Foundation develops new teaching and learning materials, encourages and facilitates more and better staff development and promotes greater responsiveness to change within higher education institutions. The Foundation works in partnership with its members and other higher education bodies to develop new approaches to teaching and learning.

In developing new teaching and learning materials, the Foundation has:

- a track record of offering customers a swift and flexible response

- a national network of members able to provide local support and guidance

- the ability to draw on significant national expertise in producing and delivering open learning

- complete freedom to seek out the best writers, materials and resources to secure development.

Other titles in this series

INTRODUCTION

This unit is designed to give a broad introduction to research so students can go on to work through the other research methods texts in this series of open learning materials. In this core unit you will come across some of the basic principles of research, as well as the terminology commonly used in research.

Session One explores why we should be concerned about research in health and social care and is designed to help you consider ways in which you can use research in practice.

Session Two focuses on the research process and gives a broad outline of the stages involved in undertaking a research study and the terminology used in this process. This includes an exploration of the potential for ethical dilemmas to arise out of research activity.

Session Three explores the research process further and considers the different approaches that can be adopted when undertaking research. The aim of this session is to help you to decide which approach is most appropriate to use when undertaking research.

Session Four introduces the various methods that may be adopted in data collection and examines the strengths and weaknesses of each approach. Consideration is also given to designing tools for data collection and the factors that should be considered in this process.

Session Five examines the process of data analysis for both quantitative and qualitative design and looks at the way the data that has been analysed may be interpreted.

Session Six, the conclusion, gives you an opportunity to test your own knowledge of research terminology and design.

At the end of the unit you will find a glossary in which we have listed the main research terms in the unit with which you need to become familiar. These terms also appear as margin definitions at the appropriate points in the text. You will probably find it useful to refer to the glossary of key concepts as you work through the sessions.

LEARNING PROFILE

Given below is a list of learning outcomes for each session of this unit. You can use it to identify your current learning level and so to consider how this unit can help you to develop your knowledge and understanding. The list is not intended to cover all of the details discussed in every session, and so the learning profile should only be used for general guidance.

For each of the learning outcomes listed below, tick the box that corresponds most closely to the point you feel you are at now. This will provide you with an assessment of your current understanding and confidence in the areas you will study in this unit.

	Not at all	Partly	Quite well	Very well

Session One

I can:

- explain the nature and benefits of research-based practice in health and social care — ☐ ☐ ☐ ☐
- identify specific areas of my practice which need to be researched — ☐ ☐ ☐ ☐
- explain the basic questions which should inform any research. — ☐ ☐ ☐ ☐

Session Two

I can:

- define the meaning of terms commonly used in research — ☐ ☐ ☐ ☐
- use an academic or professional library — ☐ ☐ ☐ ☐
- carry out a basic literature review. — ☐ ☐ ☐ ☐

Session Three

I can:

- distinguish between the differing approaches adopted in quantitative and qualitative research — ☐ ☐ ☐ ☐
- outline different ways in which data can be collected — ☐ ☐ ☐ ☐
- explain the meaning of the 'population' and the 'sample'. — ☐ ☐ ☐ ☐

Session Four

I can:

- explain the concepts of reliability and validity in research — ☐ ☐ ☐ ☐

	Not at all	Partly	Quite well	Very well

Session Four *continued*

- describe what is meant by 'indirect' and 'direct' sources of data ☐ ☐ ☐ ☐
- state the differences between the data collected in a quantitative study and the data collected in a qualitative study. ☐ ☐ ☐ ☐

Session Five

I can:

- state what is meant by the terms mean, range, median, mode, standard deviation ☐ ☐ ☐ ☐
- describe the first step in qualitative data analysis ☐ ☐ ☐ ☐
- explain the purpose of using statistics in data analysis. ☐ ☐ ☐ ☐

Session Six

I can:

- carry out a critical review of a research article ☐ ☐ ☐ ☐
- define the basic terminology used in research activity ☐ ☐ ☐ ☐
- identify why a knowledge of research is useful in my own field of study. ☐ ☐ ☐ ☐

Introduction to the unit

Introduction

This session is designed to introduce you to some key issues related to research that will be explored in more detail in subsequent sessions and units. The session begins by showing how research in health and caring professions has evolved during recent decades. Throughout the session the principles of research are explained and we consider what is meant by research-based practice and how you can apply this to your own work situation.

We will consider how interest in research has grown in the caring professions and then go on to look at ways in which research can be used in practice. Case studies will be used to illustrate some topical areas of research in health and social care.

Session objectives

When you have completed this session you should be able to:

- describe how research in the health and caring professions has evolved during the past thirty years

- explain the nature and benefits of research-based practice in health and social care

- identify specific areas of your practice which need to be researched

- define the nature of evaluation research

- explain the basic questions which should inform any research.

1: The evolution of research in the caring professions

For many years health and social care was delivered in a manner which reflected so-called 'traditional' approaches to practice. Practitioners who were questioned about why they delivered care in a particular way frequently stated that this was the way that it had always been done.

Many caring tasks would be carried out in a ritualistic manner because that was the way the task had always been done, not because it was the way known to be best for the recipient. In hospital nursing, for example, the ward routine was tightly controlled so that physical care of the patients was managed very strictly. But there was little evidence to suggest that tasks like making beds in a specific way were of benefit to patients. Furthermore, while patients' physical needs were cared for, little notice was taken of their psychological needs. This was not because previous generations of nurses did not care about such things – it was simply that the information about psychological needs was not available. Nurses and hospital social workers (then almoners) did their best with the knowledge available to them to care for their patients and clients. As the years have gone by, research findings have done much to increase knowledge and, as a result, a lot of traditional practice has been challenged (although it is not always easy to break routines and working practices that have been established over many years).

In the late 1960s and early 1970s (mainly due to American influence) professional groups attempted to change their approach to care in order to focus more clearly on the person receiving the care. It was at this time in nursing that academics started to produce papers on the process of nursing – the process approach – and many nurses attempted to move systems of care away from traditional 'task-driven' processes to ones in which the person receiving the care became the most important feature – so called 'individualised care'.

These changes gave rise to many new publications and helped to develop nursing as an academic discipline. By the 1980s the philosophy of individualised care had become apparent in the wider health and social care world and the individual rights of clients and patients were reflected in various government reports identifying changes in health and social care delivery.

However, just as the process approach was gaining in popularity, there came a change in emphasis with the government drive towards 'quality assurance'. This emphasis was developed by general managers who took over the management of health care from 'nurse managers' following the *Griffiths Report* (DHSS, 1985). Prior to this report, i.e. from the 1960s to 1985, all managers of health care were, first and foremost, nurses. They understood the nature of the work they were managing and were concerned with ensuring that everything ran smoothly in the hospital or department. There seemed to be an endless supply of money and ward managers (sisters and charge nurses) could order all the supplies they needed for patient care. If a ward sister ran out of dressings she would borrow from another ward; likewise staff would often 'help out' on another ward if there was a shortage of staff.

Following the implementation of the *Griffiths Report*, general managers were employed to manage health services and during the early days few of these managers were trained nurses, most having previously worked in industry. These new managers were therefore more often concerned with managing the budget than with the smooth running of the hospital. From the later 1980s to date, this has led to a very different ethos of care from that in the 1960s and 1970s. Money is now in short supply and ward managers hold their own budgets. Ward sisters and charge nurses are therefore restricted in the amount of money they can spend on supplies. This means that staff are also restricted in the care they give to patients because certain types of care may demand too many resources – for example, certain dressings are particularly expensive. Nowadays if a ward sister runs out of dressings she has to negotiate an exchange of goods to the same value with another ward sister.

The shift to general management during the late 1980s resulted in a more questioning approach to the care provided, and staff were forced to consider care in terms of its cost-effectiveness. Some nurses felt that individualised care was becoming lost in a system that only counted the cost of care. However, the impact of the new general management did not just affect the cost of care – quality assurance was also concerned with *standards* of care. This meant that both managers and practitioners were required to demonstrate ways in which the care they provided met certain 'standards'. These standards were negotiated by practitioners and managers and affected activities such as giving injections or suppositories, as well as many other tasks. These standards were stated in such a way as to ensure that the individual needs of patients and clients were met by the caring professions.

The current practice is for caring staff to explain to patients and clients exactly what care is to be given and the way it will be carried out. The 'standard' of care to be expected is therefore shared between practitioners and their clients and patients. If patients and clients are not satisfied that they have received the standard of care they were led to expect, they are encouraged to complain using a complaints procedure. The complaint is investigated by the manager and any practitioners found not to be adhering to set standards are called to account.

These new policies require that practitioners demonstrate the achievement of good quality care which is 'accessible', 'acceptable' and 'effective', whilst also achieving organisational goals of 'efficiency' in service provision.

As its name implies, *accessible care* is care which patients and clients can gain easy access to – a community health centre situated 20 miles away from the area it is intended to serve and without facilities for people with disabilities, for example, could not be considered accessible.

Acceptable care is that which patients and clients find agreeable. The current practice of 'mixed wards' of men and women is an example of care which some people find unacceptable.

Effectiveness in health and social care can be defined as care which is delivered in both an efficient and an acceptable manner. However, in practice this is often quite difficult to achieve because efficiency refers to delivering care at the lowest possible cost. Thus there is a conflict in the 'mixed ward' example because although this practice is efficient and can save money for hospitals, it is not acceptable to users.

We can see, then, that recent changes have made practitioners more accountable for the care they give. This accountability does not stop at practitioners though – it underpins the whole of the management and delivery of health and social care and is enshrined within changes in the management and administration of health and social care provision. The government White Paper *Care in the Community* (1989) resulted in people who were previously cared for in hospital being cared for in the community. This means, for example, that people remain in hospital for a shorter period following operations and has given rise to a need for more staff to be community based.

A proportion of the money needed to pay for health and social care has also been moved from hospital budget holders to General Practitioners (GPs). Those GPs who choose to be fundholders are now allocated a budget from the government. (Local health authorities have a responsibility to treat patients from non-fundholding GP practices.) Fundholding GPs use this budget to 'buy' the care needed for their patients from various providers – e.g. hospitals. This care may include operations or appointments with consultants. These GPs are accountable for their budget to the NHS Executive Regional Office in their area and once the money is spent, patients in need of expensive treatment have to wait until the next financial year. This has created a 'market economy' of health care in which different hospitals compete to provide the most efficient service to fundholding GPs. Hospitals which have the highest number of patients, perform the highest number of operations and have the shortest waiting lists, thereby demonstrate their efficiency to the government. These hospitals are therefore allocated more funds in the next year, which means they can buy more equipment and recruit more staff.

The differences between the 1990s system of health care and that of the 1970s and 1980s are clear. Managers who hold the budget for care provision cannot afford to provide services without clear evidence of why such services are needed, and it is up to practitioners to provide this evidence. For example, if a ward manager wishes to use a new dressing, he or she is required to cite evidence of its effectiveness to a senior nurse manager before additional funds will be released. It is this requirement for evidence to highlight the benefits of a certain treatment or type of care that makes current health and social care a 'research-based' practice. The only evidence that will have credibility with managers is that which is well researched. These changes have therefore resulted in health practitioners and managers recognising the value of research.

ACTIVITY I

ALLOW 15 MINUTES

Explain in a few lines what each of the following terms means in relation to health and social care:

1   Process approach.

2   General management.

3   Standards.

4   Market economy.

Commentary

1   The *process approach* served to promote the concept of 'individualised care'. It replaced the traditional task-driven approach with a new emphasis on the need to respect the rights and needs of the patient or client. Although a service based on client needs sounds ideal, it can be demanding of resources.

2   Just as the process approach was gaining in popularity, the *Griffiths Report* introduced *general management.* Care had to be assessed in terms of cost rather than in terms of whether it would benefit the client.This resulted in managers from industry taking over from nurse managers.

3   *Standards* are used to demonstrate that care is accessible, acceptable, effective and efficient and are used as a way of placing the emphasis back on the patient or client rather than on costs. The practitioner still has the dilemma of providing services that meet the individual needs of the client (accessible and acceptable) whilst still being efficient for the organisation. The achievement of acceptable and accessible services relies on research.

4   A *market economy* has recently been introduced into health and social care. Using this approach the government hopes that because hospital managers now have to compete for resources, they will therefore work harder and become more efficient. Although the intention of this ethic of competition is to enhance quality of care, it is debatable whether this can be achieved in a situation where care is so influenced by financial considerations.

The conflict between the need for standards and the market economy produces tensions between what is considered good for the client and what is economical for the organisation. Practitioners must therefore become research-minded and pay attention to *measuring* the effectiveness of the service delivered from both the client's and the organisation's perspective. It is this measurement of care which creates the need for research-based practice.

2:   Research-based practice

'Research-based practice' is now one of the most commonly used expressions in health and social care. Practitioners are increasingly required to support their statements about care provision with research evidence. It is no longer acceptable to assume that practices in widespread use as part of a caring routine are necessarily good. Neither is it acceptable to implement a new programme of care without first finding out what is already known about it and what has been done before – there is now a great emphasis in health and social services on not re-inventing the wheel! An example of research affecting practice is Bowlby's seminal research into attachment during the 1950s, which suggested that emotional damage could occur if children were separated from their parents for lengthy periods. Numerous subsequent research studies (including those of Robertson and Robertson (1967), Thornes (1988) and the Audit Commission (1993), examined the effects of hospitalisation on children. An appreciation of the distress shown by children led to radical changes in their institutional care, including changes in visiting patterns in hospital and a reduction in the use of children's homes in favour of long-term fostering and adoption.

In the clinical field, the influence of research findings on practice can be seen in the treatment of leg ulcers. Wound care has been the subject of much research during the past few years (Dealey, 1994). Traditional practices such as the use of Edinburgh University Solution of Lime (EUSOL) have been challenged after clinical studies measured the rate of healing following different types of treatment. More effective treatments such as pressure bandages are now being used.

The following case studies illustrate how research can alter medical practice and how practitioners can benefit from reviewing past research.

Changes in treatment for mental health problems

For many years electro-convulsive-therapy (ECT) was often used for people with severe mental illness, with many people having more than 50 treatments. Advances in the use of drug therapy for mental illness, as well as research into the long-term effects of ECT, have led to such a reduction in the use of ECT that it is now regarded as a controversial choice of treatment.

John is a Community Psychiatric Nurse interested in developing support services for people with mental health problems. In order to avoid using systems which have proved to be unsatisfactory, John needs to read recent articles on mental health support services. He can then go on to contact the authors of some of the articles to find out more about the pitfalls of developing a particular support service.

Research into cot death

Research findings suggested a lower incidence of sudden infant death syndrome (SIDS or cot deaths) in countries where babies sleep on their backs. This has resulted in a 'back to sleep' campaign and a change in policy in the UK, with midwives and health visitors radically changing the advice they give parents. **Carmel** is a Health Visitor who wants to find out two things: 'how many parents put their children to sleep on their backs?' and 'who or what was most influential in helping them to reach their decision?'. Like John, Carmel starts by finding out what has already been written on the subject. She may find that published research is already available which answers both her questions. If this is the case she may change the focus of her research slightly so that she can add to the growing body of knowledge in this area.

You can now see that without research-based practice many people would still be subjected to ECT unnecessarily, babies would still be dying needlessly, young children would be suffering both short and long-term effects of separation from their parents and people would still be suffering unduly due to the length of time needed for their wounds to heal. In addition to this human cost of suffering, there is a financial cost involved in ineffective practices. It is easy to see how a reduction in the length of an illness or healing process can result in a reduction in the need for institutional care or expensive hospital treatment.

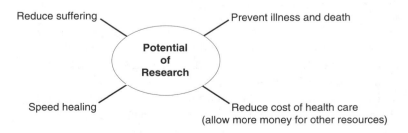

Figure 1.1: The potential of research

● your experience of using a professional library

● how successful you have been in relating research to your practice.

3: Topical areas of health and social care research

We will now consider some examples of recent research that are particularly relevant to the field of health and social care.

Research into lifestyles

We are all constantly being reminded of the importance of adopting healthier lifestyles by changing our eating habits, taking regular exercise and reducing stress levels. If you walk through the local supermarket you will see healthier alternatives to the ordinary sugar and fat-laden foods we used to buy. Health and fitness clubs have sprung up over the last few years offering a range of sporting activities to suit all ages and abilities and book shops now have more vegetarian cookery books on sale.

Until the Second World War the public was told that a nutritious diet consisted of a high intake of dairy products such as whole milk, cheese and butter. However, in the post-war years, research evidence suggested that such a diet could actually have a detrimental effect on our general health and be a major contributory factor to obesity and cardio-vascular diseases. To reduce the risk of developing such diseases, the current advice now given by health professionals is to decrease the fat, sugar and salt content in our food and to increase our fibre intake.

Another current and growing dietary concern is with the amount of additives and preservatives present in prepared foods. These can often have harmful effects on people, causing, for example, hyperactivity in children. Health visitors and midwives are now teaching new mothers different eating habits for their babies in the hope that a healthy pattern of eating established early in the baby's life will continue into adulthood.

In addition to following a healthy diet, we are also being encouraged to take more exercise because research findings have suggested a link between exercise and a reduction in heart disease. In response to this trend, health and fitness clubs have exploited the concern of the public by providing sporting activities for people of all ages and abilities. However, this increase in sporting activities has brought its own problems. For example, some people's interest in sport has developed into a fanatical interest in body building and this has resulted in an increase in the abuse of anabolic steroids (i.e. people use them to develop muscle rather than to deal with medical problems). Unusual symptoms associated with steroid use provoked an interest from medical researchers, who have now confirmed that excessive use of steroids could have tragic consequences. An obsessional need for exercise in some people has led to considerable research into the effects of exercise on the production of hormones which produce a natural 'high'.

Increased stress is another lifestyle factor which has produced a need for research. We often hear of reports suggesting that the fast pace of society has contributed to stress-related illness and this has resulted in an increase in sick leave from work. People are now frequently advised to acquire and practise relaxation techniques (for example, yoga and meditation) and to pursue relaxing hobbies.

Naidoo and Wills (1994) describe current research into lifestyles, social class and related stresses. The authors focus on factors such as income, occupational status, health inequalities, ethnic and cultural issues. Stress is not specific to any particular class or culture; it is endemic across all levels of society. Read chapter 2 of Naidoo and Wills (1994) to find out more.

ACTIVITY 4

ALLOW 20 MINUTES

1   In what ways does promoting healthy lifestyles contribute to cost saving in the economy as a whole?

2   What areas of their work could health and social care providers research in order to help people to lead healthy lives?

3   In what ways do you think health and social care providers could conduct research into the effectiveness of advice offered to patients and clients about healthy lifestyle?

Commentary

1   By keeping people healthy, fewer working days will be lost and industry will become more productive and profitable, thus contributing to the economy.

Illness is also a drain on health resources. Every consultation with a GP, for example, costs money and may result in an expensive x-ray or a prescription for an expensive drug.

Discouraging people from smoking can save resources. Smoking can result in expensive hospital treatment such as cardiac surgery or anti-cancer drugs. It may also contribute to asthma in children who then require many years of treatment. By encouraging people to live a healthy lifestyle, care providers can help to make them more productive members of society and at the same time conserve scarce health resources:

2   A few examples of what health care providers could research are whether:

●   health visitors are effective in encouraging new mothers to adopt healthy feeding practices for their children

●   weight loss programmes are effective

- health care professionals are successful in encouraging people to take regular, but not excessive, exercise

- complementary therapies are effective in reducing stress.

The social services, on the other hand, could be asking questions about, say, the quality of housing and levels of income and how these impact on people's ability to live healthy lives.

3 Here we need to consider how one measures the impact of health and social care. For example, in the case of a group of overweight people being advised to exercise more by their doctor or nurse, we would need to look at ways we can actually measure the results of taking exercise. We will be returning to this example in the next activity.

A practitioner could measure the effectiveness of complementary therapies in reducing stress by giving a stress questionnaire to participants at the beginning of the session and then again at the end of the session to find out if people feel less stressed after receiving the therapy. The practitioner could compare the effectiveness of complementary therapy in reducing stress with other methods such as relaxation or drug therapy. A stress questionnaire could be given to people who had been exposed to different types of treatment. We might conclude that the treatment which had resulted in the greatest reduction of stress was the most effective treatment.

ACTIVITY 5   ALLOW 5 MINUTES

List at least two more ways in which one could measure the physical and psychological impact of an exercise programme on a group of overweight people.

Commentary

1 One obvious way to assess the impact of the exercise programme would be to measure people's weight before and after they had undertaken the exercise programme. The comparison between the two sets of figures, or **data**, would give an indication of the *physical* impact of the exercise programme. One can normally assume that if a group of people undertake a major exercise programme this will have some impact on their weight and you might therefore expect some evidence of weight loss. However, if you have ever yourself undertaken an exercise programme simply to lose weight you will know that this cannot be guaranteed! This is an important principle in research: *what you think might happen in a given*

Data – *the information collected in the course of a research study. This may be in numerical form (**quantitative**) or in written or verbal form (**qualitative**).*

15

situation will not always happen. You therefore need to consider very carefully how you undertake any measurement.

2   You could also explore the psychological and social aspects of the programme. You could ask questions of the group, before they began the programme, about how they felt about certain aspects of life – for example, going to work or meeting other people socially. On completion of the programme you could explore the same areas. It is possible that a group of people who are overweight and generally unfit may respond very positively to an exercise programme and feel much better about themselves if they complete this programme – a psychological benefit. Similarly, if the exercise programme was undertaken in a group setting it is likely that the individual may experience some positive benefits from being with a group – a social benefit.

Whether you explore the impact of this exercise programme from a physical, psychological or social aspect, what you want to know is whether any benefits achieved were due to the exercise programme or as a result of other reasons. For example, if people report that they feel better about themselves and that they enjoyed the social experience of attending the programme, it could be that the mere *decision* to attend (taking control of an aspect of their life) is responsible for their positive feelings. For this reason it would be useful to measure the different benefits to users at *different stages* of the programme. For example, giving people a scale that measures self-esteem at different points in the programme would show whether or not a gradual increase in self-esteem can be attributed to the programme.

The relevant characteristics (or in research terms, '**variables**') of people attending an exercise programme and the way in which they could be measured are represented in *Table 1.1*. Although the expected outcome represents what one might expect at the *end* of the programme, these measurements can be made at different stages to monitor the effects of the programme throughout its duration.

Variable – *the term used to describe the characteristics or features of the objects or people in a research study. For example, variables that may be studied in relation to people are hair colour, weight, height, etc., whilst 'objects' studied could include a wound dressing, a teaching programme, a dietary regime, etc. (See also* **independent variable** *and* **dependent variable**.*)*

Variable	Measurement	Expected outcome
Weight	weighing scales	decrease in weight
Self-esteem	self-esteem scale	increase in self-esteem
Interest in appearance	interview	increased interest
Engagement in social activities	interview	increase in social life
Energy for life	interview	more energy
Amount of fat, carbohydrate and sugar in diet	questionnaire	decrease in fats, carbohydrates and sugar

Table 1.1: Measurements taken during a weight-loss programme

An understanding of research methods is important because it will enable you to identify ways in which you can monitor the impact of any care or advice you give. This example has illustrated in broad terms how one aspect of care may be evaluated and we will now go on to consider in more detail how health and social care practices can be evaluated.

4: Evaluating health and social care

As practitioners working in the field of health and social care we are interested in evaluating the effectiveness of our service delivery because, by measuring its effectiveness, we can try to determine the 'outcomes' of our care. Demonstrating effectiveness can help prove the value of what we do and thereby demonstrate the need to continue allocating resources to a given area. Attempting to prove the value of a service through use of anecdotes (such as comments from patients or clients expressing gratitude) will not persuade those purchasing care to continue buying your particular service. Moreover, it will not persuade the managers responsible for providing current health and social care systems to invest money in the future in the service you provide.

When you attempt to evaluate your work in health and social care you are undertaking '**evaluation research**'. This kind of research is not just used in health and social care – it can be used in any situation in which a service provider wishes to evaluate the success of a given service. One example might be if we, as writers of these open learning units, wanted to evaluate how well this package helps users to learn about research methods. If your experience was positive it is likely that in due course some of your colleagues would also enrol on the programme. Any comments fed back to us by users could be addressed in future editions. Your comments and those of your colleagues could provide us with a means of evaluating the success of our material.

We will now consider some situations which might have involved you in evaluating some aspect of your work or life.

ACTIVITY 6   ALLOW 20 MINUTES

Have you recently evaluated some aspect of the service you provide to clients? If so, write down:

1   Whether this was formal or informal evaluation.

2   What you evaluated.

3   The reason for your evaluation.

4   What measurements you made and how these were recorded.

Commentary

1   You could, for example, have evaluated whether your chosen method of studying this course was effective or whether a service you provided to clients in the course of your work was actually useful. It is possible that you may in the past have evaluated an aspect of your work informally without realising that you were doing so. For example, whenever you ask yourself how valuable an aspect of your service is to your patients or clients you are evaluating your work.

2   Your reasons for evaluating some aspect of your work or life could include:

   ● a desire to improve your performance to benefit users of your service or yourself

   ● a need to demonstrate in a work context your worth as part of a work appraisal

   ● a desire to confirm to yourself that something is worth doing or that your service is of a good quality

   ● a need to make future plans about some aspect of your life or work.

3   You may have made very informal measurements of this aspect of your life or work, such as conversations with friends or with other staff, clients, patients or relatives. Alternatively, in a work context you may have asked users to evaluate your service with a questionnaire which you then **analysed** and shared with your manager.

Analysis – *the process of interpreting data.*

It would be useful at this stage to share your experience of evaluating your work services with other students, colleagues or a mentor. Possible discussion areas could be:

   ● whether it is worthwhile evaluating services

   ● what can be gained by evaluating services

   ● how we can go about evaluating our services.

5:   Principles of research: the basic questions

There are three useful questions that act as a starting point whenever one wishes to carry out research:

   ● what do we need to research?

   ● why do we intend to do the research?

   ● how will we do the research ?

What do we need to research?

Taking the effectiveness of these open learning units as our example, the question of what we intend to research is quite simple. We want to know how successful and enjoyable your learning is using this package. Notice that we are not only interested in the *outcome* of your learning (measured by success), but also in the *process* of your learning (which may be expressed in terms of how enjoyable or satisfying the learning experience was). Both these factors are important elements of the 'what' question because each will require different methods of collecting data. This will be discussed further when we look at how we will do the research.

Why do we intend to do the research?

The 'why' question is essential to research. In health and social care there is little point in conducting a research project purely because you are interested in the subject or simply because you would like to increase your knowledge of the subject. These two reasons may be good from a theoretical viewpoint, but would not necessarily result in an improvement in client care. For example, finding out the *number* of different groups of people who suffer from AIDS would do little to improve the care given to these groups. To improve care you would need to focus your research on the specific *needs* of different groups of people suffering from AIDS. Clark (1987) refers to this as 'passing the 'so what?' test' – some information may generate the conclusion 'so what?' because it is not particularly useful or relevant. Referring to nursing research, Clark suggests that in order for research to be worthwhile it should:

- 'be based on a question that is relevant to patient/client care, and with potential to improve client care'

- 'yield results that are potentially either of practical value and/or theoretical significance, contributing to the existing body of scientific knowledge'

- 'be useful to other nurses as well as yourself'.

These principles could be transferred across the range of health and social care provision. If you think that the conclusions from carrying out some research in your area could generate a 'so what?' response then you need to think again about what you want to research and why.

ACTIVITY 7 — ALLOW 5 MINUTES

Which of the following case studies could generate a 'so what?' response? Give reasons for your answer.

1 Lucy is a school nurse who wants to conduct a literature review on asthma in school children so that she can increase her own understanding of the illness.

2 Dal is a diabetic liaison specialist nurse. She wants to find out what services are available for diabetics in general practices. If services are lacking she wants to improve her liaison with practice nurses in order to provide an out-reach service to diabetics.

3 Jim is a social worker who wants to study ancient history.

Commentary

Lucy would generate a 'so what?' response because she is only furthering her own knowledge base rather than specifically contributing to client care. Dal's research, on the other hand, has the specific aim of improving the service provision for diabetics. Jim's research may be very interesting and relevant to him, but will not impact on the care he is offering – he would probably not pass the 'so what?' test with his managers if he was looking for support to do research in this area, unless it could be proved to be of use in some way in his work.

The 'why?' question can also be asked about these open learning units. We can ask the question 'Why do students use open learning packages as a means of understanding research methods?' If students demonstrate success in their learning we might conclude that they use the packages because they find them effective. However, we could be drawing a false conclusion. For example, students may have had difficulty understanding the packages and have resorted to using a variety of textbooks which have given them sufficient knowledge to understand this text. Similarly, they may not have enjoyed the learning experience because they did not find the package inspiring, but nevertheless have persisted and completed the course. We would need to find out about both the *quality* (satisfaction) and the *quantity* (success) of learning in order to establish why students use open learning packages.

The question of quality is an important part of our 'why?' question in relation to this course because, when we have data about it, we could make changes to the package in response to the results of the evaluation.

How will we do the research?

The 'how?' of research is probably the most difficult because we have to choose between a variety of methods for collecting data. For example, we could evaluate students' experience of using this package by using either a questionnaire or an interview. Both of these methods have their advantages and limitations. If we sent a questionnaire some students might be too busy to return it – they might have been quite satisfied with the programme but lack of time stops them telling us that. Alternatively, failure to return the questionnaire may be because of disenchantment with the whole experience. Unfortunately, we would then not know exactly why questionnaires were not returned – a lack of response will not signify either satisfaction or dissatisfaction. As you will see in Session Four of this unit, the actual design of questionnaires is also important. It is very easy to devise questions about an experience, but it is not so easy to ensure that these questions are not biased in any way.

If we adopted another approach to evaluating the impact of our package and conducted interviews, we would then be concerned with different issues. How could we ensure that interviewees were not influenced by the interviewer and felt obliged to answer in a particular way? A student might, for example, think the interviewer only wants to hear the good things about his or her experience and so hold back on the bad aspects. This problem will also be discussed further in Session Four of this unit.

Read the case study in the box below which raises some issues of evaluation in health and social care. When you have read the case study decide upon an area for research in your own practice and answer the questions following the box.

Since the mid 1980s people with learning disabilities have been rehabilitated in the community. Some people live in sheltered accommodation, some live in social services hostels and others in small group homes. Many people have been transferred to this accommodation following years of institutionalisation - a transition that would involve a tremendous adjustment for even the most stable person. Social and health care workers now work in community settings to support people with learning disabilities. However, how can such workers know whether:

- the care people with learning disabilities receive meets their individual needs?

- the quality of life of people with learning disabilities in the community is better than when they lived in large institutions?

- staff are adequately trained to care for people with learning disabilities in the community?

- the needs of people with challenging behaviour are being met in community settings?

These are some of the questions facing practitioners working with people with learning disabilities. These questions provide the 'what' of research.

The 'why' of research is explained by the desire to enhance service provision so that the needs of clients are met in a manner which respects the right of individuals to dignity, compassion and self respect.

The 'how' of research depends on the actual research question which will be posed. For example, the adequacy of staff training could be elicited by a survey of staff which asked them about courses they had undertaken and how well these had prepared them for their role. The quality of life of clients could be addressed by using a 'quality of life' measuring scale. Several of these scales have been validated by researchers and consist of a list of items which respondents tick to indicate their agreement. The score obtained from the scale indicates the person's quality of life. However, this would only measure his or her quality of life at this particular point in time and it would not be possible to compare this with his or her quality of life before being transferred to the community. The researcher would also need to ensure that the client was actually able to understand the questions asked and would need to handle interviews sensitively.

Although providers of health and social care are interested in evaluating their services, it can be hard for them to choose from the many alternative approaches to research which could be of equal benefit to the client. Some researchers, for example, believe that one can deliver a better service by finding out first **what clients want** from the services provided. This can be achieved by conducting a survey of local users to find out what they want from services. Other researchers feel one first needs to gain a better understanding of the **behaviour of specific groups of people** in order to provide a more appropriate service for them. One cannot assume, for example, that people from different cultures, of different age groups or from different life styles will be able to make the best use of the services. One first needs to find out about the specific needs and preferences of such different groups.

1 *What area* do you think it would be useful to research?

2 *Why* would you like to conduct this particular research?

3 *How* would you like to conduct the research?

Commentary

1 Your own example will probably be from the perspective of staff working in health and social care. One example in this area might be changes in service provision which have resulted in new working practices and thus caused a certain degree of stress for staff.

2 In this instance, the 'why' is that one might want to research ways of reducing stress for staff. However, some might argue that this stress has arisen more from the pace of people's lives nowadays than from the changes in working practices. Unless we could prove otherwise we would have difficulty in arguing the case for higher staffing levels, counselling and support services for staff, or for improved in-service training programmes.

3 We could find out about stress in the staff by various means. We could examine sickness records to measure the incidence of stress-related illness or we could interview staff about what they consider to be stressful experiences. However, we could only capture the existence of stress at this point in time and would therefore find it hard to claim that this stress was a result of changes in working practices. In order to demonstrate that

stress was directly linked to changes in working practices we would need to examine staff experiences both *before* and *after* the implementation of new working practices. Such an approach to research demands careful planning and organisation – this will be discussed further in Unit Two of this series – *Qualitative Research Methodology*.

Another example could be in the area relating to services for the elderly. Services for older people have been subjected to scrutiny since the implementation of the Care in the Community Act (1989). Institutional care provided by social services departments is slowly diminishing and the private sector is growing rapidly. But certain kinds of questions still need asking, such as:

- how much notice do we take of the wishes of older people and their carers when deciding where the person should be cared for?

- do older people experience a better quality of life in their own homes than in residential accommodation?

- do adequate support services exist for carers of older people in the community?

These are important questions because the answers to them should influence service provision. Ways in which we could answer them would be by interviewing clients and carers or perhaps by using some validated measure of quality of life. We could also use statistics to ascertain whether there is a correlation between the age of the person and his or her quality of life.

Summary

1   We have traced the evolution of research-based practice over the past 20 years and looked at the social policies that have informed this development. We have considered the importance of research findings to practitioners and service providers.

2   Research can be used to:

- find out what our clients want from us

- enable us to gain a better understanding of our clients so that we can deliver a service which meets their needs

- measure the effectiveness of the services we provide.

3   Some areas that could benefit from research activity have been explored. We have briefly considered ways in which one can carry out research.

4   We have introduced the 'what, why and how' of research to enable you to consider what you would like to research, why this could be a useful area of research and how you would expect to carry out the research.

Before you move on to Session Two, check that you have achieved the objectives given at the beginning of this session and, if not, review the appropriate sections.

SESSION TWO

What is research?

Introduction

In this session we begin by identifying a suitable research problem and take you through the process of reading the literature, designing your own study, collecting and analysing your data and, finally, reporting your findings. We also discuss ethical issues which can arise when conducting research in health and social care.

Session objectives

When you have completed this session you should be able to:

- outline the process of research involved in a research study from idea to completion

- define the meaning of terms commonly used in research

- consolidate your knowledge of how to use an academic or professional library

- carry out a basic literature review

- discuss the potential ethical dilemmas that may arise out of practitioner research.

1: The research process

There is no particular secret to the research process – it is merely a systematic approach to problem-solving. Many practitioners of health and social care view the word 'research' as being synonymous with the word 'questionnaire'! The general tendency used to be for practitioners to give a questionnaire to a set of respondents, then try to make sense of the findings and subsequently present this information as a research report. Although this approach does capture the essence of research, it does not properly follow the research process. In this session we are going to look at what this process really involves. We will start by considering the problem-solving approach to a situation outside the field of health care.

ACTIVITY 9   ALLOW 15 MINUTES

Imagine that you have decided to go on holiday abroad for the first time. Write down your answers to the following questions:

1   How are you going to decide where to go?

2   How can you gather information about the country and a suitable resort?

3   What will you do if you get conflicting opinions from the information sources you use?

4   How can you check your initial information to ensure that it is reliable?

5   How will you make use of all the information you have so that you can reach a decision?

Commentary

1   You would probably decide where to go by considering a range of sources, including travel agents, libraries, the media and friends who have visited the country before. In research terms this could be described as 'obtaining data'.

2   You would gather information about the country and suitable resorts by consulting travel brochures, library books and the other sources used in Question 1.

3   If you found conflicting information you might conclude that at least one of these sources is 'unreliable' (an important concept in research), and you would need to question why this is so. Could it be that the information is out of date and the resort has changed since it was written, or was the information from a friend who has different tastes to yours?

4   You would probably check (or 'analyse' in research terms) the data you collected by cross-checking it with different sources to ensure it was true ('reliable').

5   Having assured yourself of the 'truth' value of the data you would probably search through the various accounts of the data for characteristics ('themes') that you would find attractive in a holiday resort. At some stage in this process you would probably develop a hunch ('**hypothesis**') that one holiday resort is more suitable than others. It is on this basis that you would make your decision.

In *Table 2.1* you will see a more detailed breakdown of holiday planning and a direct comparison of this with the research process.

Example in holiday planning terms	Research process
a) Decide where to go on holiday	Identify a research problem
b) Read library books/articles about holidays abroad	Find out what is known about the subject
c) Draw up a list of places/ persons from where information can be sought, e.g. travel agents, TV programmes, friends. Decide what questions to ask, e.g. weather, cost, entertainments, if vaccinations are required, type of passport required	Decide how to find more information Decide what information you need
d) Visit the places/people identified above and find out what you need to know. Make a record of the salient points	Collect the information (data)
e) Check the various sources of data against each other. Are they consistent? Find out more about any inconsistencies	Analyse the data
f) Check your findings against your original assumptions and findings. Are your findings consistent with what you found out in your first review of the information concerning holidays abroad? What explanations can you find for any inconsistencies?	Make sense of your findings
g) Decide where to go on holiday and make a list of the things you must do to ensure the holiday is a success	Reach a conclusion and make recommendations

Table 2.1: Explanation of the research process using the holiday planning example

Hypothesis – *a statement of a relationship between two or more* **variables**. *The hypothesis will always include at least one* **independent variable (IV)** *and at least one* **dependent variable (DV)**. *For example, 'eating excess calories (IV) will result in an increase of weight (DV)' (see also* **null hypothesis**).

Having completed the task in this activity you can now appreciate that we use research in many decisions we make in life. We conduct research before buying a new car or a large item of electrical equipment such as a fridge or washing machine. It would be unusual to spend a substantial amount of money before finding out or 'gathering data' about the item first.

In this example there is obviously some similarity between obtaining information from different sources about holidays and collecting information from different sources for research. The 'cross checking' that you engage in when planning a holiday also occurs in research and, as you will see in later sections, the degree to which this occurs will depend on the particular approach to research you adopt.

2: The research process in health and social care

Having looked at the process of research in relation to selecting a holiday we will now discuss the process in a health and social care context.

ACTIVITY 10   ALLOW 15 MINUTES

Read the case study below and then define the research problem. Describe the process that Brendan would go through in responding to his manager's request.

> **Brendan** is a social worker in an area of deprivation. The incidence of theft from cars and 'joy-riding' in the area is increasing and adolescents are becoming more violent. The local council has been allowed to inject some money into the area to reduce the crime rate. Brendan has been asked by his manager to investigate the need for social services provision in the area to reduce the incidence of adolescent violence. His manager wants to know what initiatives have been developed elsewhere, as well as what services the local people actually want. He has asked Brendan to submit a report of his findings which will be used to ascertain the amount of funding needed.

Commentary

Brendan has been faced with a clearly defined research problem – the types of social services provision needed in a given area to reduce the incidence of adolescent violence.

He would probably start his research process by finding out what is already known about this subject in general and what is being done elsewhere. He would therefore visit a library and read as much as possible about current services provided for adolescents.

Once Brendan has found out what is already known about the subject he would then decide how to collect information relevant to his own area. He might, for example, use a questionnaire that had been used in a different area and which was described in the literature he read. Alternatively, he might decide to interview local residents to find out how they think the problem should be addressed. Making decisions like these about how to gather this information (data) is referred to in research as the 'design' of the study.

Once Brendan has decided how to collect the information he needs, who to collect it from and what tools to use to assist him, he would then go out and collect the information. Once these data are collected he would analyse them – that is, he would count the number of responses to each question in the questionnaire or interviews so that he could get a sense of the way most people feel. He would then return to his original reading to see if there are any similarities between what he himself found and what was found by people researching in other areas. If the findings were similar he could feel more confident that his own findings were typical of the wider problem. This also means that he might be able to rely on the suggestions of other studies in solving the problem.

Having analysed the data and compared them with other studies Brendan would then be in a position to draw conclusions and present a report of his findings for his manager.

The process we have just discussed is very typical of the research process and can be described using the following headings:

1 Identify a research problem.

2 Read the literature pertaining to the problem.

3 Design the study.

4 Collect the data.

5 Analyse the data and present the findings.

6 Compare the findings with the original literature.

7 Draw conclusions and make recommendations.

8 Present a written report.

It is very important in the final stage of the research process for health and social care professionals to write a report. In contrast with the results from your research into holiday venues which have relevance only to you, there would be little point in carrying out a research project as a health or social care professional if the findings were not reported to others. In many ways this could be seen as an extension of the 'so what?' test. If you do undertake some research, but do not make your findings available to anyone, then your colleagues will probably say 'so what?'. There is clearly a need to demonstrate some outcomes from your research. We will now use the headings listed above to provide a more in-depth discussion of the research process.

Identify a research problem

In Session One we suggested a variety of issues relating to health and social care which would be amenable to research. We also mentioned that your research problem should meet certain criteria proposed by Clarke (1987) to ensure that the research passes the 'so what?' test.

When you start a research project your research problem may well be expressed in quite vague terms. At the beginning of the research process it is not always possible to be very precise because we normally do not know enough about the area of study. Examples of complex research issues which might be problematic to research because there are so many possible areas of investigation are:

● support for carers in community settings

● attitudes of health and social carers towards HIV and AIDS

● knowledge of pregnant teenagers about child care

● quality of life in community care for people with learning disabilities.

ACTIVITY 11   ALLOW 15 MINUTES

Select an area of research that you would like to carry out which is related to your professional practice. (You may wish to use the example you selected in Session One). It is important to select an area of genuine interest because you will be using your example throughout the rest of this session.

The following case studies illustrate the types of problems health and social care workers are interested in researching.

> **Kathy** is a social worker and wants to find out how children in care get on at school. She therefore frames the following research question: 'What specific problems do children in care have in attending school, and how do these problems relate to their home circumstances?'

> **Andrew** works as a health visitor in a large health centre. He wants to find out whether mothers in the local Asian community have particular difficulties in coming to the weekly child health clinic. He therefore asks, 'What factors determine attendance or non-attendance of Asian mothers at the child health clinic?'

Now write down how your particular research problem meets the requirements identified by Clarke (1987), i.e. does your research problem pass the 'so what?' test discussed in Session One?

Commentary

To check whether your problem meets Clarke's requirements turn back to the relevant section in Session One. Reread the three criteria which should be used to assess whether research is worthwhile.

Read and analyse the literature relevant to the problem

This stage of the research process requires you to conduct a literature review. A literature review is an analysis of the findings of a variety of different authors on a given subject. You may find that the subject you are interested in has virtually nothing written on it. However, don't let this deter you – you can easily broaden the scope of your subject to a related area on which more is written. (We will discuss this below under the heading 'How to conduct a literature review'). In analysing the findings of different authors we need to make some judgement about the *value* of the conclusions that these authors have reached. To be able to do this we need to compare the findings of the authors against some given criteria such as:

● the overall design of the studies

● the sample size and sampling technique

● the techniques used to collect data

● how the data were analysed

● how the results from the research were reported.

A literature review, then, is not just a summary of who said what. It is an analysis and evaluation of the findings of different authors writing about research on the same topic.

ACTIVITY 12   ALLOW **10** MINUTES

Bearing the literature review in mind, write down answers to the following questions.

1 Why do you think you need to conduct a review of the literature (including journals, books and other respected sources on your chosen subject) rather than just getting straight on with the job of carrying out research?

2 **Sandra** is a community psychiatric nurse. She has an idea for a research project investigating the impact of the recently implemented supervision register for people with mental health problems. She's keen to make a start on the research immediately until Judy, a colleague, tells her that

she would benefit from reading the literature because this will give her useful information about the experiences of other researchers. In what ways might the experiences of other researchers be useful to Sandra?

Commentary

1   The literature review is an essential precursor to the research process because, first, it helps you to be more precise about the nature of your research. You couldn't get far in designing your research project without refining your initial conception. For example, you may be interested in carrying out research into breast feeding, but unless you are more specific about what you actually want to study in relation to breast feeding you would be faced with hundreds of articles covering subjects as diverse as the nutritional content of breast milk, attitudes of partners to breast feeding and factors affecting successful breast feeding. The literature review helps you to refine your research problem into a precise question or hypothesis.

Second, the literature review informs you about what research has already been done on a given subject. By finding out what is already known you can then identify areas of unexplored territory, commonly referred to as 'gaps in the literature', which you may wish to explore in your research.

2   By reading about the experiences of other researchers Sandra can not only learn from their findings. The literature indicates how other researchers have undertaken their research, how they collected their information or data and how they managed the problems that commonly face researchers. This information will tell what has worked well and what pitfalls to avoid and will guide her in constructing her own research project.

How to conduct a literature review

Equipment for searching through the literature

Conducting a literature search can involve you spending considerable time in a library conducting either a manual or a computerised search. You may be able to obtain the help of a specialist librarian with particular interest in your field of study. Clinical school libraries are actually prepared to give free tutorials in how to do a literature search – it's part of the librarian's job. All you have to do is ring up and make an appointment with them. Even if you don't want to do this, a librarian can still help you understand how to use databases etc.

ACTIVITY 13   ALLOW 2 HOURS

The growth of computer technology has created the facility to search out information very quickly – assuming you have the skill to use this technology. If you are not familiar with the range of facilities available in your local library, it is important that you take a couple of hours to go and explore how your own library functions. After you have done this fill in the box below.

Remember that you can always ask the librarian for help.

	Available in local library	If not available there, where else?	How does it work?
Microfiche			
Database			
CD-ROM (compact disc read only memory)			
Abstracts and Indices			

ACTIVITY 14   ALLOW 2 HOURS

Now find an introductory textbook on research and read through the chapter which deals with literature searching. Clifford and Gough (1990) contains a chapter on literature searching for nursing literature. Use your reading to identify the four steps involved in conducting a literature search.

Commentary

The steps involved in a literature search are as follows:

1 Identifying key words in the research problem.

2 Selecting articles.

3 Making sense of the literature.

4 Applying the literature to your own study.

We will now look at these in detail.

Identifying key words in your research problem

This involves breaking the research problem down into key words. These can then be used as the basis of your search for information. The following is an example of a research problem.

Research problem identified: the quality of life of people with learning disabilities following rehabilitation in the community.

Notice that, at this stage, a specific research question has not been formulated and that the area of research is relatively vague. It merely states the area in which the researcher is interested.

ACTIVITY 15   ALLOW 5 MINUTES

Using this research problem, suggest some key words which you would use to begin your search. Suggest the order in which you would use these words in your literature search. This will give you a structure and help to focus the search.

Commentary

The term 'learning disabilities' is probably the first key word with which to start your search. However, you will find that, despite the fact that there is much written on this subject, it may only be possible to identify a small amount of the relevant data using this key word. This is because the term 'learning disabilities' is not recognised in American literature and the subject is referred to as 'mental retardation' or 'mental deficiency'.

If, for example, you were using a **CD-ROM** which contained the world-wide literature, you would need to key in the words 'mental retardation' or 'mental deficiency' in order to obtain the latest research. You may have the same problem with a more old fashioned database search because in Britain the term 'mental handicap' was used before 'learning disabilities'. Terms like 'special needs' are

CD-ROM – *compact disc, read only memory; an abbreviation commonly used to describe computerised library indexes of published articles and books.*

still favoured by some authors and others may use 'learning difficulties ' rather than 'learning disabilities'.

Even when you've chosen the right word your problems aren't over, because a CD-ROM machine may show hundreds of references for 'mental deficiency'. You would need to reduce the options by keying in more information. For example, you might use the word 'de-institutionalisation' for the topic 'rehabilitation in the community'. An imaginative approach can reduce the number of references to search through from hundreds to tens. *Figure 2.1* illustrates the process of choosing key words.

A list of the full references of all up-to-date research relating to your research problem can be printed out. Your next task would be to find the actual literature on the shelves or, if it is not available, to order it through inter-library loans.

By identifying key words and using them in a logical order you can save time, reduce the frustration of working through inappropriate references and keep your mind focused on the task in hand. However, you will need to be both knowledgeable and imaginative in your selection of key words.

Research question:

'What is the *quality of life* of people with *learning disabilities* following *rehabilitation in the community*?'

Key words in order in which they would be keyed in:
- learning disabilities
- rehabilitation in the community
- quality of life.

Synonyms if key words cannot be found:
- **learning disabilities**

 learning difficulties
 mental retardation
 mental deficiency
 mental handicap
 mental sub-normality
 special needs

- **rehabilitation in the community**

 relocation
 community care
 de-institutionalisation

- **quality of life**   life satisfaction

Figure 2.1: The process of selecting key words in a literature search

Selecting articles

The actual process of searching the literature can be quite time consuming. However, the degree of organisation you introduce into your research will determine the amount of time you are obliged to spend on this.

Two of the most common problems you might encounter at this stage of the research process are either a lack of articles on the subject or such a large number that it is difficult to focus the subject sufficiently to reduce the amount available.

In a situation in which there is a lack of literature you need to broaden your key words to reflect a wider area of interest. Suppose, for example, that you were interested in the role of the *practice nurse* in achieving the Health of the Nation targets set by the government in 1989. If you were unable to find any specific reference to this you would expand the search to include the role of *nurses* in general in achieving the Health of the Nation targets. You could then use this information and try to apply it to the role of the practice nurse in your own study.

The alternative problem, of too much literature, requires the reverse approach. For example, HIV and AIDS would generate thousands of references so you would need to narrow your focus considerably. Even 'women and HIV' would probably generate a good number of articles. However, if you focused in on 'counselling of HIV positive women infected by blood transfusions' the number of references would be substantially reduced.

ACTIVITY 16   ALLOW **20** MINUTES

Return to your own research problem and identify all the key words that could be used in your literature search and write them down in the same way as shown in *Figure 2.1*.

Commentary

Obviously we can't know exactly which key words you identified or how you got on with your searches, but if you had problems you should ask your tutor or a librarian for advice.

ACTIVITY 17

Visit an academic library or a professional/clinical library and, using your key words, obtain a list of about six references for your proposed area of study and then get photocopies of the relevant articles or pages. (You will need copies of these articles in order to continue working through Session Two.) If you need to use a CD-ROM machine you may need to book this in advance with the librarian.

Commentary

How did you get on? If you had any difficulties with this activity talk to your tutor.

One of the questions students ask most frequently is 'how many articles are sufficient for a literature review?' The answer to this question depends largely on the subject of the review. In the last activity we asked you to obtain six articles. However, this was only for the purposes of this exercise and a literature review for a research study would probably require more than this. Some subjects, for example AIDS, will require a larger number of articles in order for you to demonstrate that you understand the breadth of research on the subject. Of course, other subjects will have almost nothing written on them. This should not, however, deter the novice researcher from conducting a study – when published your research article could be the first of many!

Where there is no research specific to your area of enquiry you should widen your scope. For example, a search on the subject of the psycho-social impact of heart transplantation may yield only a limited number of articles, as this form of treatment is relatively new in general health care. However, the principles of all kinds of organ transplant are the same – in that they are generally a life-saving form of treatment – and so research on other forms of transplantation could provide a base from which to develop your own work. If you followed up the references given at the end of the first of your articles, you could eventually generate a reasonable breadth of knowledge on transplantation even if you didn't have any specific information on your own area of interest.

As a general rule, the absolute minimum for a reasonable literature review would be six articles; it would normally be appropriate to review considerably more than this.

Make sense of the literature

In order to make sense of the literature you will need a basic understanding of:

- research design
- samples
- the techniques used to collect data
- data analysis.

These will be discussed in more detail in subsequent sessions, but we have provided brief explanations in the following boxes to help you in the next activity.

Research design

This refers to the overall plan for collecting and analysing data. There are many ways this can be done, but for the sake of simplicity we will only refer to two broad approaches. 'Quantitative research design' refers to studies in which the researcher collects data that can be measured and summarised numerically. In contrast, 'qualitative research design' is a non-numerical approach to data collection. People participating in qualitative studies are often asked to respond to a researcher's questions in their own words and it is these words that are analysed and interpreted – the researcher does not attempt to put any numerical measure on this kind of data.

Samples

A sample is a proportion of people from a given population with whom you carry out your research. If, for example, someone asked you to comment on a sample of wine from a batch of a particular type and brand you could probably feel pretty satisfied that the taste of the wine in the rest of the batch was the same as the one you tasted – you wouldn't feel the need to taste wine from every single bottle. This is the principle behind sampling – you would interview a sample that is typical of a larger population. Of course, human respondents are not like bottles of wine – they all have different opinions and may change their minds. By giving a questionnaire to, or interviewing, just one person from a population of one hundred we can't be *certain* that their responses will be typical of all the others. We therefore need to have a sample that is as large as is feasible for the nature of the research and this is why 'sample size' is important.

We also need to ensure that as far as possible the researcher does not 'select' people to participate in the study knowing that they are more likely to respond in a particular way. This is the principle behind 'random sampling'. Using this method every person in the population being studied has an equal chance of being included in the study and the researcher has no influence over this. A less reliable method is 'convenience sampling' in which the researcher selects people who are available and agree to participate in the study. This means that the researcher has some control over the sample selection and this fact alone may 'bias' the results so that we are less sure that responses are typical of the whole population.

Techniques of data collection

These refer to all the instruments that the researcher can use to collect information. You may decide, for example, to use questionnaires and then to interview a small number of the respondents to gain a more in-depth picture of their views. Alternatively, you could observe your subjects and could either:

● write down all your observations

● video the subjects

● use a coding sheet to fill in specific categories as they occur.

If you were carrying out clinical research your methods of data collection might include blood tests, blood pressure recordings, temperature recordings, or even photographs of wounds at different stages of treatment.

When you read the literature you need to decide whether the methods selected for different studies were appropriate and whether a more accurate picture could have been gained by using additional or alternative methods.

Analysis of data

Analysis of data involves making sense of your findings from the research and is divided broadly into 'qualitative data analysis' and 'quantitative data analysis'.

Qualitative data analysis involves making sense of the data by trying to understand each specific sentence of the researcher's notes or the respondents' paragraphs written on a questionnaire. Qualitative researchers often look for themes to develop from the data which they then categorise so that they can make their findings clearer. Their data are often presented using paragraphs with quotations from interviews highlighting particular points that the researcher wishes to make.

Quantitative data analysis can be sub-divided into 'descriptive statistics' and 'inferential statistics'.

Descriptive statistics are simply a description of the findings, such as '80 per cent of the sample said "no" and 20 per cent said "yes"'. These are presented as graphs, bar charts or pie diagrams with explanations in the text explaining the story behind the statistics.

Inferential statistics are used when the researcher wants to do more than just describe the data. Imagine that your descriptive statistics show you that respondents who prefer to be referred to by their surname by health professionals also seem to be in a particular age group and a particular social class. At this point your descriptive statistics have merely provided you with a 'hunch' or 'hypothesis' about the data you have collected. Inferential statistics will allow you to apply a particular statistical procedure to find out whether your hypothesis is true (significant).

Once you have selected the relevant articles you will need to 'actively read' them in order to provide benefits for your research. Actively reading research articles requires the following steps:

1 For each article use a fresh piece of paper, record card or computer file. Write down the **full** reference for the article.

2 Write down brief notes about each article which include:

- the research problem – what the research is about

- noting whether the researcher is basing the research on any theories

- the overall research design – is it quantitative or qualitative?

- the techniques used for collecting data (e.g. questionnaires, interviews)

- the type and size of sample

- how the data were analysed

- the main findings

- any criticisms you have of the article.

3 Use your notes to generate themes from your reading. These will become the sub-headings for your literature review.

4 Under each theme compare and contrast the findings of different authors.

You may find *Table 2.2* a useful format for drawing comparisons between different authors. (You will probably need to enlarge it in order to be able to write clearly in it.)

Article	Problem	Theories	Design	Techniques of data collection	Sample	Analysis	Findings
1							
2							
3							
4							

Table 2.2 : Format for analysing research reports

5 Your comparison of different authors should also include some judgement about whether one author's work is more valid than another because of the methods used.

6 Conclude your review of the literature with a summary of the main findings and how these affect your own study.

ACTIVITY 18   ALLOW 60 MINUTES

Review one of your six articles using the six steps outlined above. This review only needs to be completed in note form, as the process of reading and making sense of what you read is most important at this stage. You may find that it takes you a lot longer than the time allocated to do this in depth, but we suggest that you initially spend only an hour on this activity and then return to the exercise later as your knowledge of research increases. You can add the detail from your other articles as you get time.

Applying the literature to your own study

The final stage of the literature review is to assess the specific value of the literature to your own study. It also enables you to become sufficiently knowledgeable about the subject for you to define the area you would like to research and to make a more specific statement about your research. You may do this in several ways. You can simply ask a question that requires an answer. So, for example, the research problem area outlined earlier:

> *'The quality of life of people with learning disabilities following rehabilitation in the community'*

could be rephrased to ask the question:

> *'Does the quality of life of people with learning disabilities improve following rehabilitation in the community?'*

Alternatively, the researcher may use literature to form the aims of the study. For example, it may be stated that:

> *'The aim of the study is to examine the quality of life of people with learning disabilities following rehabilitation in the community.'*

A knowledge of the literature can also be applied to the formulation of a **hypothesis**. This is a statement of association between the factors (or variables) involved in the research. For example, in this study the research is looking at:

- quality of life (variable)

- people with learning disabilities (variable)

- rehabilitation in the community (variable).

Any hypothesis will comprise at least one 'independent variable' and at least one 'dependent variable'. The dependent variable is so-called because it 'depends on' the independent variable. The independent variable is so-called because it is not dependent on any other variable and is manipulated by the researcher. The administration of a drug is a good example of an independent variable because the researcher can 'manipulate' the dose. The dependent variable would be the effects on the patient because they depend on the drug.

A hypothesis might state:

> *'The quality of life of people with learning disabilities will improve when they are rehabilitated in the community.'*

ACTIVITY 19

ALLOW 2 MINUTES

State the 'independent' variable and the 'dependent' variable for the above hypothesis.

Commentary

The 'independent' variable is the *rehabilitation in the community* because this can be manipulated by the researcher – the researcher can compare the experiences of people who live in the community with those of people who still live in hospital.

The 'dependent' variable is *quality of life* because it *depends* on rehabilitation in the community. It cannot, therefore be manipulated by the researcher.

ACTIVITY 20

ALLOW 15 MINUTES

Think about and write down a research question for the research area you identified earlier.

Commentary

Look at your question and decide whether it is clearly stated as an unambiguous question, or whether it is a vague research problem.

So far in working through the research process we have covered:

1 identifying a research problem

2 reading the literature pertaining to the problem.

We will now go on to the third step.

Designing the study

We will be exploring issues relating to research design in more detail in Session Three but for the moment we will discuss how research design shapes the research process as a whole and how this relates to your proposed area of study. As you will recall, 'research design' refers to *how* the study is carried out – and the way in which you carry the study out will depend on *what* you want to know.

When you ask a research question you need to think how you are going to get the answers to that question. This will involve collecting information which describes the situation that exists at present. You might, for example, ask people with learning disabilities how they feel about being in the community after being in an institution.

Obviously the extent to which you will be able to gather this information will depend on the degree of disability of those interviewed. You may need to consider who else would be in a position to comment on this situation and you may conclude that the social and health care staff of the community homes would be key people to ask, as would the families and friends of the people with learning disabilities. If you were to collect data from all of these groups by asking them questions, your approach to research would be described as a 'descriptive study' – you are simply describing what is going on.

Once you understand the principles of a descriptive study it becomes easier to understand the difference between a research question and a research hypothesis. In asking a question you are not seeking to change the situation in any way in the course of your research – you are simply asking the question and collecting information to help you to find the answer.

In the hypothesis stated above we have suggested that there is a relationship between the quality of life and living in the community, stating that the quality of life will *improve* as a result of living in the community. Therefore when planning our research design to explore this hypothesis we need to consider *how* we can demonstrate that this relationship exists.

In this case we need to collect information about how the different groups identified above feel about care in the community because that will tell us how they feel *now*. However, this will not tell us whether the quality of life of the people with learning disabilities has improved. To be able to state that with any degree of confidence we would need to know about their quality of life *before* living in the community. We would therefore need to gather information about our group of people with learning disabilities both before and after they had moved to the community.

Collecting information before and after the change to community care would enable us to compare these two sets of information or data to see whether the quality of life has improved. This approach to research is known as 'experimental design' because, unlike the descriptive approach, there is some *manipulation* or *change in circumstance* that is being measured. Just as the researcher can manipulate an experiment by choosing how much of a drug to give, the researcher in this case can choose to study people both before they are discharged into the community and after they have been rehabilitated. It is this change in circumstances (administration of a drug or rehabilitation in the community) that constitutes an experiment. So, in considering our research approach, we need to decide whether we are going to undertake a 'descriptive study' or an 'experimental design'.

There is one other aspect that should be considered at this stage. That is the way in which you are going to collect the information.

ACTIVITY 21   ALLOW 5 MINUTES

List two ways in which you think you might collect information for research.

Commentary

1   You may have suggested that you could ask people to answer your questions, either by giving them written questions to answer or by personal interview where you ask the questions face to face.

2   You can also collect information by watching or observing what is happening.

These two methods represent the most common means of data collection and we will be looking at these in more detail in Sessions Three and Four below. You may have also noted other ways of collecting information such as looking at records and accounts of experiences.

The next decision to be made concerns the *kind* of information or data you will collect. Again, this is fundamental to your research design. You might collect data in a very structured way such as using a questionnaire which has a number of questions that demand one-word answers such as 'yes' or 'no'. If you collected this kind of data from several people you would then simply count up the number of people who had answered 'yes' and the number of people that had answered 'no' to your question and base your results on this finding. This process of organising your data numerically is called 'quantifying your results' and consequently these data are commonly described as **'quantitative data'**.

Alternatively, you may wish to ask more open-ended questions in your interviewing or by using a questionnaire. The difference in this approach would be that instead of asking people to respond to a highly structured questionnaire with pre-determined answers such as yes or no, you will be asking them to respond in their own words. This produces 'qualitative data' because it is data expressed in the respondents' own words. The focus is on the *quality* of the data produced, not the quantity.

So, to use our example of care in the community, if we gave the staff caring for people with learning disabilities a questionnaire that contained a lot of questions demanding a fixed response we would be collecting quantitative data. For example, we might ask if they feel community care is better for this client group and ask them to indicate 'yes' or 'no'. If, on the other hand, we ask them to describe in their own words how they felt the care of this group was influenced by being in the community we would be generating **qualitative data.**

We will be discussing **research design** in more detail in the following sessions, but before we do that we will continue our journey through the research process.

Research design – *refers to the overall plan for* **data** *collection and* **analysis** *in a research study.*

Collect the data

The next stage of research is the data collection stage. When planning your research you need to be quite specific about how you are going to collect the data. As you will see in Session Four, this includes a need to consider the actual mechanics of data collection, such as how you might give out questionnaires and collect completed forms.

ACTIVITY 22   ALLOW **15** MINUTES

Returning to your own research idea, think briefly about how you would design your proposed study and how you would collect your data. (At this stage we are only concerned with a very broad overview, so do not spend too long on this activity. We will return to this area at a later stage for a more in-depth review).

1   State what kind of design you think you might use to answer your question – descriptive or experimental.

2   State how you will collect the data.

3   State the kind of data you will collect – will it be qualitative or quantitative?

Commentary

Now that you are beginning to think seriously about your research it would be a good idea to discuss your intentions with other students, colleagues or a mentor. In particular, you should discuss your research with a tutor to ensure that you are on the right track.

Analyse the data and present the findings

Once the data have been collected the next stage of the research process is to analyse them. The analysis of data can be divided into three methods, depending on the type of data collected. These three methods will be dealt with in more detail in Session Five but are introduced briefly here.

As discussed above, quantitative data will be in a form that allows you to organise your data numerically using statistics. (We will be exploring ways of managing numerical data in more detail when we discuss statistical approaches.) The important point to remember here about statistics is that their purpose is to summarise a set of numbers in a meaningful way.

Descriptive statistics – a type of statistics used to describe and summarise data. For example, the data from a research study may be presented in percentages as a means of summarising large sets of data (see also inferential statistics).

We can use a very simple kind of statistics known as 'descriptive statistics' to summarise our data. Although many people are fearful of statistics when they approach research for the first time, it is useful to remember that we all actually use statistics on a daily basis. For example, if we heard that an opinion poll had suggested that 80 per cent of the population preferred a particular brand of chocolate we would not panic and try to understand what this meant – we would recognise this as a claim that the majority of the population held this view. Such a statement is an example of descriptive statistics. Descriptive statistics literally describe the data – for example, the number of respondents who answered 'yes' to a particular question or a percentage of the sample who strongly disagreed with a statement on a questionnaire.

Sometimes, however, it is not enough to simply state the basic facts. This is where the second type of statistical analysis can be useful. We might want to draw some conclusions from the data so that we can comment on the wider implications of our research. You will remember from our previous discussion of 'making sense of the literature' that **'inferential statistics'** involve statistical procedures which tell us whether or not our hypothesis is true. They are called 'inferential' because they 'infer' some type of cause and effect.

Using an earlier example, inferential statistics might confirm our hypothesis that people of certain age groups and social classes are more likely to wish to be referred to by their surname by health professionals than people from other age groups and social classes. Also, returning to our example from the field of learning disabilities, inferential statistics might show that people with learning disabilities who are rehabilitated in the community score significantly higher on a quality of life measuring scale than those who remain in hospital. Don't worry if the idea of inferential statistics seems rather complex at present – we will examine it in more detail in Session Five.

The final type of analysis we need to consider is what we would do with 'qualitative' data. Here we are dealing with words rather than numbers and so we have to look at different ways of analysing the data. The effort here is organised around looking at the words generated by the research to try and derive common patterns or themes in the data. For example, if the people in the learning disabilities study were asked to describe how they felt about community care, a number might give positive comments about a certain aspect of their experience – such as their increased social life – and we might then identify this as a common theme in our data. Again, we will be exploring this further in Session Three.

ACTIVITY 23 ALLOW **10** MINUTES

Think about your proposed area of research and state which of the types of data analysis you think you will be likely to use.

Commentary

It will be useful to compare your approaches to data analysis with other students, colleagues or a mentor. It is also worthwhile seeking a tutorial with your tutor at this point. As you will see in Session Five, the sooner you think about how data from a particular study can be analysed the better.

Compare the findings with the original literature

The final three stages of the research process are much easier, although just as important as the earlier stages. Once you have analysed your data it is vital that you compare your findings with those mentioned in the literature. You may have noticed in published works that a brief review of the literature appears early in the article, to be returned to later in order to demonstrate whether it is supported or refuted by the author's work.

Draw conclusions and make recommendations

The conclusion and recommendations are a vital part of any research project. It is the recommendations that service providers are most interested in. If your recommendations are balanced and framed constructively there is a good chance that they can be used to justify changes in practice. Of course, service providers will also be looking for flaws in your research. However influential your recommendations may be, they will not inform future practice if the sample size was too small, if your questionnaires were poorly designed or if the research was biased.

Present a written report

Presenting the written report is often the point at which novice researchers run out of steam! A clear and succinct report with strong recommendations is more likely to be disseminated by your employer to other relevant parties than a vague summary would be.

A research report should ideally include the following:

- a title

- an abstract (a brief, concise summary of the main points)

- an introduction indicating the research question and the purpose of the research

- a literature review

- a research design

- data analysis and presentation of findings

- a comparison of the findings with the original literature

- conclusions and recommendations.

3: Other issues to consider in planning research

Before we move on to the next session there are a couple of other issues that must be explored. These include a consideration of how researchers go about getting permission to undertake research and how the potential ethical dilemmas generated by research are resolved.

Permission to do research

Refer back to the problem area or research question you set yourself at the beginning of this session and consider who is going to be involved in your research. If you wish to study any group of people who form a group because they belong to a specific organisation you will need to think about how you will get access to them. You may, for example, wish to ask students on a health and social studies programme about their views of changes in health and social care provision. To do this you would need to approach the course leader in the first instance. He or she would advise you of any procedures you must follow to get access to this group of students. The same principle applies if you wish to study a group of patients in a hospital setting or a group of elderly clients in a residential home. You must get permission to access this group from the person responsible for the area. This may seem a rather cumbersome process but there are several good reasons why it should be followed.

First, it is a matter of simple courtesy to request access for the purpose of research. This applies even if you actually work in the areas where you might be planning to do some research. Second, there are legal requirements linked to data protection that limit the access of unauthorised persons to data about individuals. Legislation entered within the Data Protection Act 1984 prevents unauthorised persons accessing data about individuals. The Act safeguards sensitive personal data and contains internationally agreed principles that guide the use and storage of data on computers.

Finally, as the range of research in health and social work increases, a manager might be the only person who has a clear insight into the number of times a particular group is being asked to participate in research.

Imagine that these units of study on research methods represented a revolutionary new approach in the education of health and social workers using distance learning. A number of people might be interested in researching the impact of this new method of education. If access to you as a student was not managed by one person it would be possible (as, indeed, has happened in the past) for you to be inundated with researchers asking for help in their study of educational programmes! While you might be very willing to participate the first time, enthusiasm tends to wane after the third or fourth questionnaire or interviewer arrives. In such a situation there would be a risk that you might not comply with the study or you might give inaccurate data because you are weary of answering questions. The problem of access can be a real problem for many managers working in specialist areas of health and social care delivery.

Even when permission has been granted to approach members of a group in an organisation, this does not guarantee that the researcher will get the data they want. You may have the full support of a manager to ask staff in a unit to participate in your research, but the staff themselves must also have the right to refuse and, indeed, commonly do so!

Ethical issues in research

Permission to proceed with a study in any organisation involving health and social care usually carries the prerequisite that the proposed work has been scrutinised by an ethical committee – to ensure it does not have the potential to cause harm in any way to the participants.

All research projects, no matter how small, must be approved by a local ethics committee. It is your task, as the researcher, to demonstrate that any ethically questionable issues involved in your research are necessary in the pursuit of knowledge and potential improvement in client care. Ethical issues are mainly concerned with a balance between protecting the rights of people for privacy, safety, confidentiality and protection from deceit, whilst at the same time pursuing scientific endeavour.

Ethics committees have been established for many years in health care. These committees are made up of groups of experts in health and social care who have expertise in both research methods and health care. Committee members include doctors, nurses and lay members and other members of the health care team as required. The purpose of ethics committees is to protect the interests of the public. Research in health and social care is becoming so widespread that there is a danger that members of the public may be subjected to insensitive questioning techniques, or even the collection of information from them for which they have not given informed consent.

Procedures for submission of research to ethics committees vary across the country. You need to contact your manager or the committee secretary in the first instance to find out the procedure in your own area. The frequency with which the local ethics committees meet varies between areas and you will need to bear this in mind if you wish to submit a proposal for ethical approval. Normally, a researcher will be expected to submit a *summary* of their proposed research to the ethics committee on a form supplied by the committee.

ACTIVITY 24

Imagine that you are the subject in the following research scenarios. In each case write down whether you consider it to be ethical or unethical.

1   You have been asked by the head-teacher of your teenage daughter's school if you would be willing to allow her to complete a questionnaire on 'relationships' for the school nurse. You ask to see the questionnaire and find that one of the questions is 'Which of the following types of contraception would you use?'

2   You have agreed to participate in a drug trial requiring you to give a blood sample (after you have starved for twelve hours) every week for eight weeks. The first and last blood tests are to be taken from your veins. The tests in between will be finger prick tests. When you attend for the second finger-prick test the research states that these tests have proved unreliable and so full blood tests from your veins will be required in all the six remaining tests.

3   A student has been allocated to you for a two-week period. You regularly have students placed with you and are required to teach her the basics of your job. At a later date you discover that the 'student' was really a researcher who was using participant observation to collect her data. Her research focus was the experiences of students in placements in health and social care settings.

4   You are approached in your local shopping centre by an undergraduate student who wishes to ask you some questions about lifestyle. She says she is interested in the diet people eat, the exercise they take and the use of strategies to reduce stress. After agreeing to answer some questions the focus of the questionnaire moves rapidly through diet and exercise and on to personal relationships at work and at home. You suddenly realise that you are revealing the most intimate details of your life.

Commentary

Obviously you will have subjective reactions to these scenarios. This illustrates the fact that ethics in research is a complex issue. One could argue that research is *never* truly ethical because subjects are always inconvenienced in some way. We need to consider at what point inconvenience could threaten someone's safety. In the case of the blood test, for example, it could be a major inconvenience and, indeed, unsafe to fast for twelve hours on a regular basis. Furthermore, using full blood samples rather than finger-prick tests could make some participants feel temporarily unwell. But the researcher might argue that this study is of sufficient importance and benefit to the common good to make the inconvenience worthwhile.

This illustrates the ethical dilemma in research. If we were to be truly ethical all of the time it would not be possible to advance our knowledge through research. Perhaps a better measure of whether or not research is ethical would be whether the subject is *harmed* in some way rather than being inconvenienced. However, 'freedom from harm' is difficult to define as there are a number of situations in which subjects might not be harmed physically, but could experience psychological harm – from insensitive interviewing, for example.

ACTIVITY 25   ALLOW 15 MINUTES

Look again at the scenarios in the last activity. Which do you think might have the potential for psychological harm? Give reasons for your answers and suggest ways in which such harm could be reduced.

Commentary

Scenarios 1, 3 and 4 could all cause psychological harm, although scenario 3 is probably the least harmful of the three.

In scenario 1 the school nurse is making assumptions about sexual activity in school children and could be seen to be condoning sexual activity. Teenagers not engaging in sexual activity might feel that they ought to be and could feel 'abnormal' as a consequence.

Scenario 4 could be very harmful as the interviewer could easily touch upon sensitive areas and might cause considerable psychological damage. Furthermore, interviews of this nature shouldn't be conducted in a shopping centre and require a skilled interviewer who is able to handle questions in a sensitive manner.

Scenario 3 is probably less harmful, although you might feel pretty angry if you found that your movements had been observed and recorded during the past week. You might wonder what use is to be made of the research findings and you might be worried because there were days on which you did not perform at your best. You might also be concerned about the anonymity and confidentiality of the research.

It is very important to ensure that anonymity, confidentiality and privacy are maintained in your research. As far as anonymity is concerned, you can only be sure that your participants are anonymous when even you, as the researcher, are unable to link information with the participant. Clearly, in observation research and interviewing this cannot be achieved. It is therefore of utmost importance in these situations to assure the participant that the findings will be totally confidential and will be used for the purposes of the research only.

Participants should also be assured of confidentiality by researchers trying to gain informed consent. The term 'informed consent' means the participant has been fully informed of the nature and purpose of the research. The participant is unlikely to give consent if the research seems to be of a dubious nature. In face-to-face situations the researcher is able to explain to the participant in detail about the importance of the research, and is therefore more likely to gain their co-operation. In questionnaire surveys, however, the researcher must rely on a covering letter to explain the research. The letter needs to be brief, but convincing enough to persuade the respondent to take the time needed to complete the questionnaire. Lack of attention to covering letters can result in a poor response rate to questionnaires.

However, gaining consent also brings difficulties in that if the participants have information about the research it may influence their behaviour. This is most likely to occur in interviews and observation research, but can also occur in questionnaire surveys and, to a lesser extent, in experiments.

Various problems arising from the issues around gaining consent are illustrated in the four scenarios above.

In scenario 1, when the researcher explains the nature of the research, he or she might unwittingly present certain attitudes – perhaps authoritarian or tolerant – and this could affect the responses of the teenagers. You might think, therefore, that in order to avoid the effects of researcher bias it would be better for the participants not to meet the researcher. However, this course of action could be considered unethical because the participants might not then have given their informed consent. One could argue, however, that by the very act of completing the questionnaire the participants are giving their consent. Nonetheless, most ethical committees would consider that such consent had not been given in an informed manner.

Scenario 2 is a good example of how a subject can give informed consent to one procedure, but then be exposed to an alternative procedure. In this instance informed consent should again be sought when the procedure is changed, a new consent form should be signed and care taken to ensure that the subject does not feel coerced into continuing with the study.

Scenario 3 illustrates the problems involved in observation research which arise when the researcher is trying to avoid a situation where the participant behaves differently because of the presence of the researcher. Because the researcher wishes to gain a 'warts and all' picture she cannot make the subject aware of her research but she must, however, always maintain utmost confidentiality about what she observes.

Scenario 4 illustrates the importance of participants fully understanding the nature and purpose of the research project. When asking respondents to complete a questionnaire clear information must be provided and respondents given a choice of whether to 'opt in' or decline. In this situation the respondent was placed in a position where she misunderstood the nature and purpose of the research and as a consequence faced questions that appeared not to match the stated intention. It could be said that the undergraduate student had been unethical in this case.

Before we conclude this session one final activity will help you to apply ethical considerations to your own research.

ACTIVITY 26   ALLOW 10 MINUTES

1   Think about your own proposed research project which you identified earlier. Write down any ethical implications which might arise in connection with your research and how you intend to deal with them.

2   Find out the procedure for submission of research proposals to ethics committees in your area of work. Your line manager will be a good place to start. Also, find out how long it takes to get approval for a research project.

Commentary

Since we cannot comment on your particular project it is a good idea to contact your tutor or mentor to discuss your research plan before you submit it to the ethics committee. Ethical committees have become more stringent in their rulings since the growth of research activity in health and social care during the past twenty years. You will therefore need to build sufficient time to gain ethical approval into the time-scale for your research. You also need to be aware that ethical committees can reject a proposal for research on its first submission for a variety of reasons, including:

- risk to patients/clients
- lack of sufficient information about how the research will affect participants
- poor evidence to indicate that confidentiality will be assured.

In addition, the committees will comment on poor research designs, particularly if they put people at risk.

Summary

1 The research process we have outlined in Session Two illustrates the 'what', 'why' and 'how' of research.

2 The 'what' of research corresponds to the identification of a research problem.

3 The 'why' of research can be likened to a review of the literature pertaining to the problem.

4 The 'how' of research corresponds to designing the study, defining the sample, collecting, analysing and presenting the data.

Before you move on to Session Three check that you have achieved the objectives given at the beginning of this session and, if not, review the appropriate sections.

SESSION THREE

Research design

Introduction

Having explored some of the general principles of research, we will now consider in more detail the different approaches that can be adopted when designing a research study in health and social care. We will explore the approaches of quantitative and qualitative research and consider the important issues relating to sample selection in research.

Session objectives

When you have completed this session you should be able to:

- distinguish between the differing approaches adopted in quantitative and qualitative research

- describe what the term 'triangulation' means

- outline different ways in which data can be collected and analysed

- explain the meaning of the 'population' and the 'sample'

- outline the ways in which samples can be determined in both quantitative and qualitative design.

1: Research design: ways of approaching research

Various dictionaries define research as a 'careful search or inquiry', a 'process of systematic investigation' or 'a course of critical investigation'. Underpinning all of these definitions is an emphasis on a structured, organised approach to finding out information.

Some definitions refer to a 'scientific study' which implies a very specific approach to finding out information. It has been noted elsewhere (Clifford and Gough, 1990) that the use of the word 'scientific' may serve to confuse as it carries with it associations of working in a laboratory – a world very distant from the world of work of many health and social care professionals. However, references to 'science' in research are sometimes used to indicate a particular orientation in the way research should be conducted, usually implying the quantitative approach (which we will return to below).

The way in which research is approached is commonly referred to as the 'research design'. This term refers to the overall plan for deciding how the information or data will be collected and analysed. It is this overall plan that governs the approach the researcher will take in the study. We will now consider these various approaches.

2: Quantitative and qualitative research

There are two broad schools of thought on how research should be conducted. Both represent different ways of finding out about the world around us. In many research texts these different approaches are frequently defined as quantitative and qualitative approaches to research. You have been introduced to these ideas in the previous session and we will now elaborate on what they involve.

Although using these two words to define approaches to research is somewhat simplistic, it is a useful way of drawing the distinction between differing schools of thought. When research is referred to as having a 'quantitative orientation' it implies there is some form of factual relationship between the data collected. In contrast, in qualitative research the emphasis is on the 'quality' of the data collected rather than the quantity. We will go on to look at exactly what these terms mean in the next activity.

ACTIVITY 27　　　　　　　　　ALLOW 30 MINUTES

Read the two case studies presented below and then list the ways in which the approaches that Stephen and Lesley have taken to their research differ.

> **Stephen** is a new social worker who has been assigned to work in a busy inner-city area. There has recently been a change in boundaries for the social services and, as a result, when Stephen tries to map out his potential client group he finds that he has not got an up-to-date record of the spectrum of clients he might meet in his new job. He decides he will establish this data by undertaking a small study in

which he will seek to find out a number of things about his area. He wants to find out about the age range of the people in the area, the type of housing, the average income, the number of people employed and unemployed and the number of people with disability. He plans to collect this data from records available from the census that was completed in the previous year. This gives him access to a large amount of information about clients in his area and he can work out from this a picture of the potential client group he will be working with.

Lesley is a community nurse whose client group includes a small number of people who are suffering from cancer. Lesley is concerned that she does not know enough about how these clients feel about having cancer and therefore cannot help them as well as she would like to. She decides that the way to improve her knowledge is to undertake a small research study in which she interviews a few of her patients about how they feel about having cancer.

Commentary

The ways in which the two case studies differ can be summed up as follows:

1   Stephen wants to collect a lot of *factual* information about a large number of people. He wants to identify facts in numerical form so that he can determine the numbers in each group.

   Lesley wants to collect information about how a small number of people feel about their condition. She does not intend to gather a lot of facts, but wants to know what it means to people to have cancer.

2   Stephen knows exactly what data he wants to collect.

   The kind of information Lesley collects might be quite wide and varied – she does not know what her patients will say to her about their condition.

3   Stephen can collect the data he wants fairly quickly from existing records.

   Lesley might take quite a long time collecting the information through interviews.

4   Stephen does not intend to collect his data by face-to-face contact with his potential client group. He is going to access records that have the detail he wants.

Lesley will be directly involved in collecting data from the people she meets in her work.

So, we have noted a difference between the *type* of data that is collected and the *volume* of data that is collected. Did you note all these points? If not, read the case studies again now and look out for them.

Our two case studies above illustrate the main differences between quantitative and qualitative research. Quantitative research is an approach to research that relies on:

- *objectivity* – the researcher collects data in a way that is distant from practice

- *'hard' data* – that is, data which can be measured and quantified in some way

- *statistics* – the results from studies following the quantitative approach to research are presented in numerical form and are interpreted on the basis of the statistics calculated.

So, for example, if Stephen analyses his data by age group he would be able to identify how many people in each age group he had in his locality. In this case he is using a numerical figure to indicate what he has found in this part of the data collected.

Quantitative research represents what might be described as a traditional view of science – that is, measuring hard data and accounting for results in statistical terms. To be able to do this in a sound, reliable way the researcher using quantitative methods must ensure that the data collected is objective and not biased (we will look at the topic of bias later on).

Quantitative research is a 'deductive' approach to research, in which the researcher starts with something they know a little about and want to explore further. In our example above, Stephen knows about the variables of lifestyle, such as age ranges, patterns of employment and so on, that he might find in society. What he wants to find out is how this is reflected in his own locality.

In qualitative research the researcher is searching for *meaning* in a given situation and therefore collects data in the *form of words* – the medium by which most of us normally explore meaning. So, for example, Lesley wants to hear from the cancer patients so she can understand their needs. This is known as an 'inductive' approach to research – the purpose of the research being to find out what the patients think and to bring that knowledge into view. The inductive approach seeks to generate ideas rather than to test existing ideas.

ACTIVITY 28   ALLOW 5 MINUTES

Think of an example of each approach which could be used in your own work.

Commentary

Check your answers with a mentor or tutor to see if you are on the right lines.

3: The research continuum

It is useful for the newcomer to research to realise that experienced researchers often have strong views about their own particular research orientation and may view quantitative and qualitative approaches to research as mutually exclusive. This has resulted in many commentaries and articles from both sides criticising each other's approaches. However, as we will be demonstrating in this unit, both quantitative and qualitative approaches to research can provide useful data in social and health care research. Rather than seeing these approaches as mutually exclusive it is perhaps better to view them on a continuum as illustrated in *Figure 3.1*.

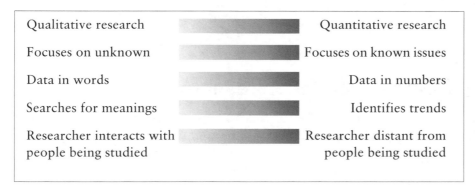

Qualitative research	Quantitative research
Focuses on unknown	Focuses on known issues
Data in words	Data in numbers
Searches for meanings	Identifies trends
Researcher interacts with people being studied	Researcher distant from people being studied

Figure 3.1: The research continuum

In *Figure 3.1* we have listed the key features about each approach that have been noted so far, but rather than present them as polar opposites we have shown that they can lead one from another. For example, a researcher might ask people to say in their own words what they felt about how the government was managing the country today. People might say: 'I think they are doing a good job', or alternatively, 'I do not think they are doing a good job'. The researcher might end up with data that contains many similar responses and so might note the results to this question as '50 per cent thought the government was doing a good job and 50 per cent thought the government was not doing a good job'. Although this researcher collected qualitative data he or she has to some extent expressed the results in quantitative terms.

Triangulation – *the use of more than one method of collecting or interpreting data. For example, using* **observation** *and* **interviews** *or structured* **questionnaires** *and* **interviews**.

Triangulation

Another reason for not preserving the idea that quantitative and qualitative studies are mutually exclusive is that, in many studies, people will use a mix of them both in their approaches to data collection.

We might, for example, be planning to undertake a qualitative study that consists of asking open questions about a particular problem area. However, when doing this we might also want to collect some quantitative data about the individuals we are studying to help us to understand the situation a little more. For example, in the case study above, Lesley is clearly taking a qualitative approach to her data collection in trying to identify how people feel about having cancer. However, she might decide that she also wants to collect some factual data about her clients, such as their age, gender and occupation, as this might help her determine whether these factors make a difference to how they cope with the disease. If she did this she would be collecting data using both quantitative and qualitative approaches.

If this idea of mixing approaches is developed further and a researcher decides that he or she would collect data *on the same problem* in a number of ways this is known as triangulation. Triangulation is the use of more than one method of collecting or interpreting data. So if Lesley was going to use triangulation with her patients with cancer she might collect data by both observing and interviewing them. This way she is focusing on the problem from two angles – by watching people and by talking to them. In so doing she might observe that people with cancer look unhappy and anxious and, when asking them how they feel, might find that her interviewees tell her they feel unhappy and anxious. If this was the case then her conclusions from her observations would be supported by her findings in the interviews. She can state that the overall conclusion from her study is based on more than one perspective. The value of triangulation, therefore, is that it is a means of validating conclusions based on one perspective.

4: Data collection in research

In order for research data to be capable of being quantified it must be collected in such a way that it lends itself to quantification. When planning how to collect the data researchers therefore need to consider whether the approach they are intending to use will enable them to quantify or count the responses. In qualitative research a more open approach is required which allows respondents to tell it in their own words. Here, the researcher is less concerned with being able to count the responses and more concerned with being able to record in words what the respondents have said.

Whichever approach is used, the tools or techniques employed in data collection are questionnaires, observation and interviews. We will be returning to the topic of techniques for data collection in Session Four, but it is useful at this stage to clarify some terms relating to the use of data collection tools.

Some questionnaires, for example, are described as 'highly structured' – meaning that they carry a fixed range of responses which enable the researcher to calculate the number of people that respond to each section quickly and rapidly.

Interviews can also be highly structured. You may, for example, have been approached in the street by someone undertaking a market survey exploring your views on a particular brand of product. In this case you will probably have been asked to give a single response only to questions relating to brand preference.

At the other extreme you may be faced with a 'low structured' questionnaire which asks you to describe in your own words what you feel about a situation. This is obviously an approach more suited to qualitative research design.

Figure 3.2 shows some illustrations of questions using both a high and a low structure.

Highly structured questions

Do you smoke?   *Yes* ☐   *No* ☐

How many cigarettes do you smoke each day?   0-5 ☐ 6-10 ☐ 11-15 ☐

Should health risks associated
with smoking be taught in schools?   *Yes* ☐   *No* ☐

Low structured questions

Please state your views on cigarette smoking.

Please tell me what you think about health education in schools.

Figure 3.2 : Illustration of different question types which can be used in questionnaires or interview schedules

We can use the same principles of high or low structure with observations in research. For example, if we wanted to undertake a study designed to measure the workload of care assistants in residential homes we could begin by listing every task care assistants carry out in their work. We could then observe care assistants at work and record the frequency of each task and the time taken for each task. *Figure 3.3* shows an example of how you might do this.

Alternatively, if we were using a low structure in these same observations we might start our study with a much more open approach and simply divide the categories of care up into those involving direct contact with residents and those that do not involve direct contact. The researcher in this instance would write down in some detail the nature of the task and any other observations relating to it. *(Figure 3.4)*

Area of work	time	time	time	time	time	time
Walks with resident to toilet						
Helps resident wash						
Serves meal to resident						

Figure 3.3: High structure observation schedule

Working directly with resident

Task:

Comment:

Not working directly with residents

Task:

Comment:

Figure 3.4: Low structure observation schedule

We will now look at data collection in quantitative and qualitative research in more detail.

Data collection in quantitative research

Quantitative research is useful for researchers from a variety of perspectives:

- as a worker in a health care or social setting you might want to provide information about your workload

- a health visitor working with a group of first-time mothers might wish to calculate the particular needs of her clients against those required by another group of clients in another district

- a social worker might want evidence to prove that he has a greater number of people with mental health problems in his area than colleagues in other parts of the city.

In these examples the data produced is of potential value in helping the health and social care professionals plan their work.

ACTIVITY 29 ALLOW **10** MINUTES

List three more examples of situations in health and social care where it may be useful to collect quantitative data.

Commentary

You may have thought of some of the following:

- client or patient turnover
- number of clients on a list
- workload measures
- success rates for complex surgery
- comparisons between the effectiveness of drugs
- gender and age mix of clients
- number of people who smoke.

Using quantitative data

Our working lives today are frequently influenced by quantitative data. However, it is useful to make the distinction between those areas where quantitative data influences your work in a managerial sense and those that impact on the care you might give. For example, if you have managerial responsibility for any aspect of care you might be asked to provide statistics to indicate the number of people working in your area or the number of clients or patients that are cared for over a given period of time. In contrast, quantitative data relating to the nature of the care you give might require statistics about outcomes of care. The demand for such statistics is illustrated by the increasing number of measures of medical care now being published regularly in newspapers – such as how many people have undergone operations for particular problems, how long they stayed in hospital and so on. It might well be useful for you to think about how you could use quantitative data to help measure outcomes in your own work.

As a further illustration of the potential use of quantitative research let us consider the number of visits by elderly people (over 75 years old) to a GP's surgery over a 12-month period. The purpose of the study would be to identify periods of the year when elderly people demonstrated a higher incidence of ill health. *Table 3.1* presents this data in simple statistical form. We have used descriptive statistics to summarise this data – that is, we have described the number of patients who have visited the surgery each month. We have also indicated alongside each set of figures what the number of visits mean as part of the overall total (of visits by elderly people to the doctor during the year) in terms of percentages. Percentages are a very common way of presenting descriptive data. We will be returning to the use of statistics in research in Session Five, but for the moment it is useful for you to see the ways in which data from quantitative research can be presented.

Month	Number of cases visiting the doctor
January	50 (10%)
February	70 (14%)
March	55 (12%)
April	50 (10%)
May	45 (9%)
June	35 (7%)
July	25 (5%)
August	15 (3%)
September	30 (6%)
October	25 (5%)
November	45 (9%)
December	45 (9%)
Total	500 (100%)
Key: percentages represent the percentage of total visits by elderly people to their GP during the year	

Table 3.1 : Number of elderly people visiting the GP surgery

We can see from *Table 3.1* that the highest number of visits by elderly people to the GP was in February. At that time 70 elderly patients visited the doctor. This represented 14 per cent of the total visits by this group of clients to the doctor during the year for which the data is presented – and there may be a number of reasons for this level of attendance.

ACTIVITY 30   ALLOW 5 MINUTES

1 List some reasons why there was a larger number of elderly people attending the GP's surgery during the winter months.

2 What might the implications of this pattern of visits be for health and social workers?

Commentary

1 The rise in attendance at the GP's surgery in the winter months can probably be attributed to the greater number of coughs and colds at that time of the year. It might also be due to increased falls by the elderly on icy roads.

2 This clear indication of increased visits by the elderly during the winter months can be useful to the doctor, the nurse or the social workers when planning services. For example, if a review of services had resulted in reducing the number of staff in the surgery the results of this study would indicate that it would not be a good idea to cut back services in the winter. The data may also indicate a need for health and social services to work closely together during this time to try and reduce the demands on resources. For example, vulnerability to infections is commonly associated with a poor nutritional state and a poor nutritional state may occur as a result of inadequate income. A GP may be able to treat an infection, but can do little to help the economic condition of those people attending the surgery. The social worker would not be able to help the infection, but would be able to identify people who need and might be eligible for additional financial support.

Limitations of quantitative design

From *Table 3.1* we made some assumptions about the underlying reasons for the patterns identified in the data. However, these assumptions could well be incorrect because, for example, one of the results of introducing a health-oriented model of health care in recent years has been that GPs have been encouraged to offer medical checks to elderly citizens as a means of promoting healthy living. The GP surgery considered in *Table 3.1* may have decided because of staff holiday patterns to introduce a health check clinic in January. If this was the case then the reason for the rise in visits could be completely different to that identified earlier.

You therefore need to remember that whenever you are reviewing data that has been generated by research you should always check to determine whether the data is sufficiently complete to enable you to draw conclusions from it. In *Table 3.1* the data on its own provides only a limited amount of information – you would need to have some more data to be able to build up a picture of the factors influencing the frequency of visits to the GP.

We will discuss data interpretation more specifically in Session Five, but for now it is useful to emphasise the point that while a set of figures can give a useful indication of patterns, if taken in isolation from the context to which they relate they can be misleading. Professional workers wanting to plan service provision to meet the needs of the population identified in *Table 3.1* would need a lot more detail about this group before they could begin.

We will now look at a published study which illustrates how researchers might carry out a research study about a health and social care issue.

ACTIVITY 31　　ALLOW 30 MINUTES

Read the article by Rita Howard in Resource 1, which explores the reasons for older people attending accident and emergency (A&E) departments. Then carry out the following tasks:

1 Make notes on how the researchers collected data for this study.

2 Describe how the researchers present the results from this study.

3 Identify any conclusions the researchers reach which would be of use to the hospital managers.

Commentary

1 Data were collected from the patients' casualty cards and by follow-up telephone interview. The authors do not report specifically on how the data were collected and recorded. However, we can assume that data from the records were quantitative because the researchers used as a focus for their study specific reasons for admission, categorised under medical categories. Similarly, we can assume that the telephone interviews were low structured as it would not be easy to use a structured approach with this medium. We must nevertheless stress that we are only making assumptions – the authors do not give direct information on their data collection methods.

2 The results are reported in some detail in a written account which enables us to read about the specific problems and reasons why older people attend A&E. This is supported by a chart *(Figure 1)* which attempts to summarise the entire written report.

3 This paper has good utility value for the hospital in which the research was located. By identifying patterns of attendance the researcher was able to identify areas where it might not be a good use of hospital resources for the older person to attend a hospital A&E department. She was able to make recommendations on the basis of these data for the future management of services to help improve the system. Obviously it would be up to the managers in the locality to decide whether they were in a position to adopt the recommendations, and it is likely that before they would be willing to undertake such a major organisational change they would require further information. They might, for example, decide to locate a GP facility within the hospital department in order to measure how much this deflected patients from the main A&E department.

Data collection in qualitative design

Whilst the quantitative approach to research has many uses we know that it is not possible to answer every question which arises in research using this approach. For example, an area of interest relating to the visits by elderly people to a GP surgery might be to identify the factors which influence the elderly person in deciding to visit the doctor in the first place – i.e. what makes them decide they have a problem. When these less specific questions are being asked then the qualitative research approach is the best one to take.

Approaches to data collection in qualitative research are such that whatever technique is adopted will be low structure. If researchers wished to undertake a qualitative study they would need to ensure that the questions which were asked allowed respondents to answer in their own words. Since in qualitative research it is more common for the researchers to try to interact with the people being researched, they would be more likely to interview people or use observation than to use questionnaires. In both cases they would still use a low structure approach.

ACTIVITY 32

ALLOW **10** MINUTES

Referring back to the data presented in *Table 3.1* try to identify three issues where quantitative data might not give a researcher sufficient information about:

a) why more elderly people visit their GP in February than in any other month of the year

b) how elderly people are received and treated by the general practice staff.

Commentary

Your examples might include the following:

- what old people feel about visiting the doctor in the winter
- whether old people come to visit the doctor because there is no other accessible service such as a health visitor or practice nurse
- how people feel about waiting in the surgery
- what social factors cause some people to visit the doctor more frequently.

As you will recall from the case study of Lesley, the community nurse studying cancer patients, qualitative research is concerned with seeing things through the eyes of the person being researched. It uses an inductive approach which seeks to generate ideas rather than to test ideas in the deductive way used in the quantitative approach. Qualitative research is designed to address questions which look for meaning and insight. We will now look at a research report which uses qualitative design.

ACTIVITY 33

ALLOW 30 MINUTES

Read the article in Resource 2 by Stephen Firn and Ian Norman on the psychological and emotional impact of receiving an AIDS diagnosis. Then carry out the following tasks.

1   Make notes on how the data were collected.

2   Describe how the results of the study were reported.

3   Explain why the researchers adopted this approach to data collection in this study.

4   List the themes identified by the researchers.

Commentary

1   The data were collected using tape recorded interviews – a common approach in qualitative research design. The interviews were focused around two questions which were used according to whether the interviewee was a patient or a nurse.

2   The researchers stated that they had identified themes in the data and were reporting on these. They did not attempt to count the number of responses in any way, but simply reported on trends that emerged in the interviews.

3   It is likely that this approach to data collection was adopted because of the nature of the subject being studied. AIDS remains a sensitive area to research and to try and identify emotional reactions through the use of structured questionnaires could be considered an inappropriate way to approach sufferers and carers. The research notes that other types of study have not adequately addressed the issues.

4   In this research report the researchers identified five main themes arising from the data:

- reactions to critical events related to HIV infection

- changes in body images and chronic ill health

- fear and rejection: the social construction of AIDS

- cognitive and minor dysfunctions associated with HIV

- absent friends: the death of loved ones through AIDS.

Using qualitative research

One reason for doing qualitative research is to begin studying areas where there is no research available – to begin the process of unearthing knowledge. The paper used in the last activity demonstrates another reason why a qualitative research design may be useful. In this report the authors noted that previous studies had failed to find out the extent and range of mental health problems experienced by people with HIV. Although some work had been undertaken, no real conclusions had been reached. Given this situation, the study in Resource 2 is useful for health and social workers because it raises issues and increases our awareness, both of which will help when working with people with HIV.

Limitations of qualitative design

Researchers advocating the qualitative approach suggest that attempts by quantitative research to place people in neat little boxes for research purposes do not reflect the real world. However, if we wanted to assess the popularity of a chocolate bar and to be able to claim data were representative of the wider population, we could more easily do so using a quantitative study than a qualitative study. We could obtain data from a larger number of people using a highly structured interview than we could using unstructured methods.

5:   Quantitative and qualitative design – choosing an approach

You are now at a point where you can apply your knowledge of quantitative and qualitative design to addressing particular research problems.

ACTIVITY 34   ALLOW **10** MINUTES

Look at the list of research questions below and write beside each of them which would lend themselves to:

a)   quantitative research design

b)   qualitative research design.

Research questions:

1 What is the incidence of accidents in under 5 year olds in the inner cities?

2 Why do some people become drug addicts ?

3 What is the relationship between income and type of housing?

4 What is the incidence of post-natal depression in one GP surgery?

5 What is the overall annual success rate in exams held in a College of Health Studies?

6 What does it feel like to be the client of a social worker?

7 What does it feel like to be a schizophrenic?

Commentary

Your answers should look like the list below. We have highlighted the key words that give you a clue to identifying the most suitable research design.

1	What is the **incidence** of accidents in under 5 year olds in inner cities?	quantitative
2	**Why** do some people **become** drug addicts?	qualitative
3	What is the **relationship** between income and type of housing?	quantitative
4	What is the **incidence** of post-natal depression in a particular GP surgery?	quantitative
5	What is the overall annual **success rate** in exams held in a College of Health Studies?	quantitative
6	What does it **feel like** to be the client of a social worker?	qualitative
7	What does it **feel like** to be a schizophrenic?	qualitative

Understanding the principles of qualitative and quantitative research is essential to understanding research. We will therefore use this final section to check your understanding of the previous activity.

Think carefully about what you have read so far about both approaches to research and then complete *Table 3.2* with the characteristics of each approach.

Characteristics	Qualitative Research	Quantitative Research

Table 3.2: The different characteristics of qualitative and quantitative research

Commentary

Your completed responses should be similar to those in *Table 3.3*.

Characteristics	Qualitative Research	Quantitative Research
Deals with known or unknown issues	Focus on the unknown issues	Focus on known issues
Type of data	Words	Numbers
Aims	Searches for meanings	Identifies trends
Researcher's role	Researcher interacts with people being studied	Researcher distant from people being studied
Structure of data collection	Low structure	High structure
Form of data analysis	Words	Numbers

Table 3.3: The different characteristics of qualitative and quantitative research

Now that we have looked at the ways in which you might collect data we need to look at how you decide *who* to collect the data from. We will explore this topic in terms of populations and samples.

6: Population and samples

Population – *indicates the entire set of subjects in a given group that could form the focus of a study. For example, all people who own television sets could be a population (see sample).*

It is important to be able to distinguish between what researchers call a 'population' and a 'sample' as these are two fundamental concepts in research. A population is all the possible occurrences of one particular variable, whereas a sample is just a smaller group comprising an element of that population. In other words, the sample is a representative of the population.

Suppose the government launched a campaign in England to encourage children in their first year at secondary school not to smoke. The population in this case would be *all* the children in England whose ages lay within this age group. Ideally, in order to test whether the campaign had been a success, one would have to question all the children in this group. However, this is clearly totally impracticable. Therefore a smaller number of children, i.e. a *sample*, would be selected and, based on the results of that sample, a conclusion would be drawn about the total population of children in their first year at secondary school.

Before we look at ways in which we identify samples we need to consider why researchers consider it acceptable to use a sample rather than the whole population. The first thing to note is that when we define a population for research we need to be very specific about what we mean. Throughout this text we have referred to 'health and social care workers'. However, there are many categories of health and social care workers including nurses, physiotherapists, occupational therapists, speech therapists, dieticians, doctors, social workers and probation officers. We could also extend the term even further to include all the support staff that work in health care to ensure the services run smoothly. Within this group each professional will have their own speciality area of practice – there are many different kinds of social workers all with their own speciality interest. It is quite likely that the views held by social workers on some aspects of care would be different to the views held by nurses. Consequently, if we simply said we were doing a study in which the population was health and social workers people reading the study would not be very clear about who exactly we were referring to.

The more specific we can be about the population that we intend to study, the more confident we can be that a sample drawn from that population will give us a representative view of the whole population. For example, we could decide to undertake a study of nurses who have been qualified for between five and ten years and who are now working in the speciality of child care. This gives us a clear 'sampling frame' from which to draw our sample. (A sampling frame is representative of the population that we are going to study.) Other sampling frames might be a group of nurses, a group of social workers specialising in elderly care or a group of patients who went through a rehabilitation programme in a particular hospital during the year 1995.

To further illustrate what we mean let us assume a group of researchers wants to study the progress of patients in a hospital. This hospital is a regional centre offering wide-ranging rehabilitation services to all people in that area who have been victims of accidents or disease. The client group undergoing rehabilitation will range from children who have been in road traffic accidents through teenagers and adults who have received head injuries, to people of varying ages who have got chronic illnesses affecting their mobility and elderly people who have suffered from strokes. The population of people who have undergone rehabilitation in hospital X is rather too broad for this research study since, for example, we know that the way children respond to care is quite different from the way adults respond. Consequently if the researchers working at this hospital wanted to establish a study they would need to devise a much more specific sampling frame from which to work.

Not only do we need to be specific in defining a sample group, but we also need to consider the issue of variables.

ACTIVITY 36   ALLOW 5 MINUTES

Let us imagine that the researchers wanted to study how effective the hospital's rehabilitation service was for people who had suffered a stroke. What kind of factors do you think they will need to consider when assessing how well stroke patients have been rehabilitated?

Commentary

The factors that may influence how stroke patients respond to rehabilitation would include:

- gender

- the age at which the person had the stroke

- how disabled he or she was as a result of the stroke

- family support at home.

You might have thought of other factors to add to this list. The important point here is that all of these factors could influence the way in which each individual responds to the rehabilitation treatment. This list of factors would be some of the known 'variables' in our study. A variable is any factor that varies within a population being studied.

Because all these factors could influence the way the person with the stroke responds to treatment, the research team would need to be very specific about the criteria they use when determining their sample. They might decide to define 'inclusion criteria' for the sample as:

- male or female patients
- aged 65-75 years
- who had the stroke within the last 12 months.

The research team might also decide that they would include people who were not too disabled and who were able to understand the nature and purpose of the study. They may also decide not to take initial account of the level of family support the stroke victim had at home, but to consider this variable when analysing their data.

Sample procedures in quantitative research

The way in which samples are collected in research is a crucial feature of research design. There are several ways of doing this. Some of the standard procedures are:

- simple random sampling
- stratified random sampling
- cluster sampling.

These approaches to sampling are all used in quantitative research. (We will outline these before going on to consider the sampling procedures used in qualitative research.) The key point in quantitative research approaches is that the sample should be representative of the population being studied.

Simple random sampling

This is the simplest form of sampling and works on the principle that every member of the chosen population has just as much chance of being selected as another member of the same population.

To take a sample using this procedure, you first need to acquire a list of every member in your chosen population. For example, if you were going to study the smoking habits of children in a particular school you would need to get a list of all the school children in the chosen population.

The next step is to draw a sample from the population at random. This could be done by drawing names out of a hat, using a blindfold or selecting names at random from the population list. However, there are more formal procedures available to assist researchers using this process. For example, if the population is particularly large, a number could be assigned to each member of the population. The researcher could then refer to a random sample table listing numbers (which can be found in many statistical books) to identify which members of the population will be drawn into the sample. An example of a random sample table is shown in *Figure 3.5*. The researcher using such a table would simply choose numbers by selecting a column from the random sample table. Alternatively, there are computer programmes available which can be used to generate random numbers. Those numbers can then be matched with those people on the list and those people would constitute the sample to be studied. (This is rather like the process adopted in the National Lottery.)

3	67	89	56	45	83	21	43	8	9	12	43
65	87	18	4	65	90	36	25	17	29	56	39
34	87	93	21	65	23	61	5	3	98	12	31
23	67	87	43	21	9	81	33	72	44	18	23

Figure 3.5: Example of a random sample table

Stratified random sampling

This is a variation on the simple random sampling technique described above. It is used when the researcher wants to divide the population into sub groups to obtain a greater degree of representation of each sub group. For example, when defining a population to study school children's attitudes to smoking the researchers may wish to study children of various ages as they feel that attitudes can change a lot with age. So, rather than selecting a simple random sample of the whole population of school children, they divide the population into 'strata' or sub populations incorporating, say, four groups; children aged 8–10, 11–12, 13–14 and 15–16 years. A simple random sample from each of these groups could then be selected.

Cluster sampling

This form of sampling involves selecting small units of a population and then using every member of these smaller groups in the research study. For example, consider a study in which the researcher wished to look at people's views about the waiting time for admission to a National Health Service (NHS) hospital for treatment. A sample of 1000 people could be selected at random. However, as this sample would need to be scattered widely all over the country it would be an expensive way of finding a sample.

An alternative approach would be to identify various NHS hospitals and view those who are on these hospitals' waiting lists as clusters of people within our sampling frame – that is, they are waiting for NHS treatment. From this collection of clusters four hospitals could be chosen at random. Then, every patient on the waiting list in each hospital could be approached (if the hospital wasn't too large) and asked for his or her view.

You may, however, realise that we have not given every NHS patient a chance to participate in this study and so are failing to follow the principles of random sampling. When we report the results from this study we must therefore note this. Researchers recognise that the data from cluster sampling will not be as reliable as that from random sampling, but it is nevertheless still a useful approach.

As another example, imagine if a group of nurses working in a newly built private hospital were selected as a cluster in a study of nurses' views on their working conditions. It is likely that the views of this group would differ from those working in an old NHS facility. This illustrates that selection of clusters is important to the research process.

The above three methods are the most widely used sampling techniques. There are, however, two others which are used in which the samples are not entirely selected at random. The first of these is called '**quota sampling**' and is mostly used in the field of market research. Here, the researcher has prior knowledge of how many participants are required in the sample group with previously specified traits (e.g. fifty females attending a health centre between the ages of 18 and 25) and will collect data from this range until the quota is saturated. If you meet a market researcher undertaking this kind of sampling approach you might see him or her ticking a list to indicate that you fall into a specified sampling group. For example, he or she might only need to interview one more person who was in the age group of 20-25 year-olds and you might come along and be the last person to fit that age group. If you were the last person in that age range that he or she needed to interview, the next person who came along in that age range would not be involved in the study.

The second alternative is '**convenience sampling**'. This is by no means an ideal method of sampling since it is not a random process. However, if time and

Stratified sample – *a technique in which random sampling can be used to select people from two or more strata of the population independently. For example, a researcher completing a study of midwives could incorporate the views of junior and senior midwives by selecting a random sample from each of the two groups, rather than selecting a random sample from an overall population of midwives.*

Cluster sample – *a sample identified as a smaller group within the larger* **population** *being researched.*

Convenience sample – *a sample from a population selected on the basis of its accessibility to the researcher rather than on the basis of random sample procedures.*

75

resources are limited this method is acceptable provided that its restrictions are stated quite clearly at the onset of the study. In this method researchers know the population they wish to study, but have constraints placed on them in terms of identifying a sample from that population. For example, a researcher who wishes to study children's smoking habits might only have a couple of months in which to collect data if he or she is doing this work in a limited time period. The researcher knows that the ideal would be to collect a random sample from the population of school children but does not have the time to meet these criteria. He or she decides instead to select a sample of convenience from just one school where subjects are readily available. When writing the report the researcher will note that the limitation of the sampling means that the results cannot be generalised to the population as a whole, but that, nevertheless, these results might indicate local trends and could be used as a basis for further enquiry.

Sample size in quantitative research

With regard to how large a sample size should be, the general rule is that the degree of accuracy required will be reflected in the sample size. (There are various ways of calculating the ideal sample for a study which involve using statistical tests. The procedures involved in this are discussed in the companion unit *Inferential Statistics* (Clifford and Harkin, 1996).

You can make judgements about the reliability of research by considering both the method of sampling and the sample size.

ACTIVITY 37   ALLOW 5 MINUTES

Look at the two research studies described below. If you were looking at the findings from the two surveys which do you think would provide the most 'reliable' information?

a) A researcher administered a questionnaire to a random sample of 1000 people.

b) A researcher administered a questionnaire to a convenience sample of 30 people.

Commentary

You would probably find the information from research study (a) to be the most reliable because the researcher has collected data from a random sample – that is, a sample that represents the population as a whole. In selecting what is a large random sample the researcher here can say with confidence that the results are representative of the population being studied and can therefore *generalise* the findings to the whole population. However, it is the fact that it is a random sample rather than the fact that it is large which contributes to its reliability.

In example (b) the researcher has selected a sample of convenience and whilst the findings might be an acceptable conclusion about that group, the researcher cannot claim that her findings apply to the population as a whole.

In summary, the question of what constitutes a good sample is quite a difficult one to define in quantitative research. As a general rule it has been suggested that a sample of at least 30 is necessary for statistical testing (Hicks, 1990).

Sample procedures in qualitative research

As you know, the purpose of qualitative research is to understand meaning in given situations. Here we are not as concerned with looking at representative groups as we are in quantitative research and therefore sampling is approached quite differently.

Looking again at our example of school children and smoking, there may be sufficient data available to indicate the number of school children who smoke and to suggest an association between smoking and other factors – for example, parental smoking habits. However, we may want to understand why some school children choose to smoke whilst others from similar backgrounds do not. In this case we wouldn't need to target a random sample of school children to look at smoking patterns overall because we already know about this problem. What we want to do is to find some children who smoke and to talk to them about it. This is called '**purposive sampling**' – the sample is selected purposively on the basis of a particular variable that is being studied, which in this case is smoking. Some authors of quantitative texts refer to this as '**theoretical sampling**' – the sample selection is driven by the theoretical basis of the study.

Sample size in qualitative research

In qualitative research the researcher looks for meaning in the data rather than to be able to generalise the findings to any wider situation. Consequently the sample size in qualitative research is generally much smaller than that used in quantitative design. It is not uncommon for research reports of qualitative studies to report on very small numbers of respondents ranging, for example, from 6 to 10 respondents. When you read qualitative research reports you will see that researchers refer to 'saturation' of data. What this means is that when deciding how many people to involve in a qualitative study the researcher will continue to collect data until the ideas that are developing are saturated – that is, no new data are being collected. So our researcher wanting to ask children about why they smoke will continue to approach new children for interviews until the same information keeps recurring.

Summary

In Session Three we have explored the differences between quantitative and qualitative research design. You should now be in a position to:

1 Define a question for research.

2 Select an appropriate research design to answer the question.

Before you move on to Session Four check that you have achieved the objectives given at the beginning of this session and, if not, review the appropriate sections.

SESSION FOUR

Techniques of data collection

Introduction

In previous sessions we have considered the issues in research design to do with collecting and analysing data. We have explored quantitative and qualitative approaches to research and looked at why studies in quantitative research are approached in a highly structured way and in qualitative research in a low structured way. In this session we will focus on how data are actually collected – the techniques available for data collection. We will, however, start by considering the issues of reliability, validity and bias that can arise when collecting data for research.

Session objectives

When you have completed this session you should be able to:

- explain the concepts of reliability and validity in research

- recognise situations in which bias can be introduced into research design

- describe what is meant by 'indirect' and 'direct' sources of data

- outline how one uses observation and asking questions as means of data collection

- state the differences between the data collected in a quantitative study and data collected in a qualitative study.

: Concepts of reliability, validity and bias in research

'Reliability' and 'validity' are concepts commonly referred to when undertaking research. Before we consider how to develop techniques for data collection it is important that you understand these concepts . The quality of a study is enhanced by the degree of reliability and validity achieved in it. However, as with other aspects of research, the extent to which it is possible to achieve them depends on whether the research design is quantitative or qualitative.

Reliability

So, what do we mean when we talk about reliability? The answer is that reliability is *'the extent to which a tool can be relied upon to give results that are consistent'*. This means that similar results would be obtained if the same test was carried out on more than one occasion under the same conditions. We would, for example, need to be able to ensure that a questionnaire administered in a quantitative study is reliable.

When a test is reliable, the results of it are completely independent of the researcher, the sample and the method used – so that no matter who conducted the test, the results would remain unaltered. The results would be more or less identical if a different sample was selected or the technique of administering the test was adjusted in some way. For example, imagine that a researcher has devised a tool to measure the stress levels of health and social care workers. If this tool was a reliable measure of stress in this group, it could be expected to yield a similar range of results regardless of whether it was administered in the north or south of England or whether it was distributed by postal questionnaire or in a group setting during a health and social care workers' study day.

There are certain useful techniques commonly applied to determine the reliability of a method. One is called the 'test-retest method' whereby the same test is carried out on several occasions and the results are then compared. So, for example, our researcher in the example above might administer the stress questionnaire to a group of health and social workers at the beginning of a month. The same test would then be administered several weeks later to the same group. If the questions were 'reliable' it could be assumed that they would yield the same results at both points in time from the same sample group. Any questions that proved unreliable could be removed from the stress questionnaire after the second test. For example, a question in a questionnaire might be phrased as follows:

Do you prefer the new treatment to the old one?   Yes ☐   No ☐

The first time the questionnaire was administered a number of respondents may have answered 'yes' to this question. If the question was reliable the researcher might expect that when it was administered the second time the same respondents would give the same responses. If they did not give the same responses it could be assumed that there is a problem with the question and that it needs to be reworded. (However, researchers should be aware that a change in response may be due to a change in opinion.)

The test-retest method is only appropriate in quantitative studies. It is more difficult to ensure reliability in a qualitative study.

ACTIVITY 38   ALLOW 5 MINUTES

Why you think it is more difficult to ensure reliability in a qualitative than in a quantitative study?

Commentary

In a *qualitative* study it is harder to develop a tool for testing the reliability of data collection because the nature of the questioning is much less structured. This means there is more scope for interviewer and respondent interaction – a factor that will have a major impact on the way in which a research tool is used. With a different set of interviewers and respondents there could be different answers to the same questions.

Validity

In research the term 'validity' means the extent to which the tool used in a research study actually measures that which it is designed to measure.

One of the reasons why it can take a long time to develop a questionnaire is that it is difficult to design a study that has questions which clearly focus on the area of study. For example, if you were going to develop a questionnaire about stress where would you begin? If you wanted to ask people if they 'felt stressed' they might answer 'yes' because simply by asking the question you have put the thought into their minds. This is why many questionnaires do not seem to ask questions directly relating to the topic of study. For example, many questionnaires on stress do not directly ask people if they feel stressed – rather they ask people whether they are sleeping or eating well, on the basis that if people respond 'no' to such questions they can be said to be exhibiting signs of stress.

Validity is a difficult thing to establish – if we are using a structured questionnaire how can we be absolutely sure that we are measuring what we are supposed to be measuring? Broadly speaking, a research instrument should have both 'internal' and 'external' validity. Internal validity refers to a situation in which the instrument measures what it is supposed to measure. So, if we refer to our example of developing a questionnaire for stress we could only say that it was a valid instrument if we were confident that our measures were actually examining the concept of stress. External validity is the extent to which our research tool would lend itself to other settings. Would our stress questionnaire 'work' if we gave it to several different groups – for example shop workers, health workers, social workers? If it was a valid scale of stress measurement then it should. Obviously, if the research tool has failed the reliability test then it won't be valid either.

There is an important variation in reliability and validity between quantitative and qualitative research. In quantitative research researchers can hope to achieve high reliability because they use highly structured tools that will be consistently interpreted each time they are used. However, because qualitative research uses low structure tools it cannot claim such a high level of reliability (since each respondent may give a different response).

However, with validity the reverse is true. It is hard to develop a valid questionnaire with high structure for the reasons noted above in relation to writing questions that will yield consistent responses. When undertaking a qualitative study it is much easier to ensure that questioning is directed towards the specific area of interest and is therefore valid. Validity is said to be high in qualitative studies.

Bias

There is always a risk when a researcher undertakes a study that he or she will introduce bias into their study. For example, a researcher who feels convinced that a particular form of treatment is the 'best', and decides to undertake some research to prove this, is starting out with the wrong attitude. This kind of approach can mean a study is biased at the outset, because the researcher is simply looking for ways to prove his or her case. This is an extreme situation and one unlikely to occur with most experienced researchers. However, it is also possible for bias to creep into research studies inadvertently at several stages. For example, a poor questionnaire design can result in bias if the questions prompt answers in a particular direction. Questions can be phrased in such a way that respondents feel they ought to agree with them, such as 'isn't it true that this is the best treatment?'

The way in which one can determine whether or not bias has been introduced in a study is by carrying out the process of critical reading of research. We will be exploring this further in Session Six.

2:   Gathering data

Researchers can gather information or data from a number of sources and these can be identified as 'indirect' or 'direct' sources. The former refers to situations where the researcher makes use of existing sources of data to collect information. The latter involves collecting data directly from people involved in a study. We will now deal with each of these in more detail.

Indirect sources of data

Indirect sources of data are sometimes referred to as 'secondary sources'. A secondary source indicates that the data have not been collected directly by the researcher, but are already in existence from another source.

We have already seen a good example of using data from a secondary source in the work you did on the study in Resource 1. In that activity you were asked to identify how the researcher (Howard) had collected the data. We noted that, initially, data were collected from the patients' casualty cards. Howard did this to check what specific problems patients came with to the A&E department and it proved a useful way of collecting data relatively quickly. If Howard had had to rely on asking all the patients attending the A&E department what their specific medical problems were it would have taken a very long time to collect the same amount of data.

ACTIVITY 39   ALLOW 5 MINUTES

List any occasions when you have referred to secondary data to help you in your work or in your studies.

Commentary

You might have been able to make quite a long list. For example, if you have been reading research reports you could categorise these data as secondary materials – they have not been collected by you and the source lies with someone else.

Alternatively, you might have consulted official statistical materials to help you in your work. Stephen, the social worker, for example, used census data to help identify factors relating to his clients.

You may have undertaken the same approach as Howard yourself in identifying from patient or client records the type of caseload you are working with.

Another area where secondary sources of data are used very commonly is in the development of auditing systems in health and social care. Frequently the main source of data available to anyone reviewing systems of health care is secondary data. It is this which is used when publishing patient outcomes following medical treatment.

Although we have highlighted several advantages in using indirect sources of data, they do also have some drawbacks. Often the data available in secondary sources have not been collected in the particular way that you need them. For example, you might be interested in finding out the number of elderly people who were admitted to residential homes over the winter months in one particular year, but the records which exist already only show you the annual figures. Similarly, you may be concerned with the number of males who were treated in a hospital for smoking-related diseases, but the figures you are given only state the total number of people treated with these diseases, regardless of their gender.

In some situations we may have no choice but to rely on secondary sources. For example, if we wanted the amount and type of data that Stephen the social worker needed, it wouldn't be possible to replicate the census, which is a major national survey sent to all households in the UK every 10 years. In this case you would have little choice but to rely on those data. However, we can at least make a distinction between the kind of data that are collected by tried and tested methods and those which come from a less reliable source. For example, patients' care records in hospital can cause difficulties in terms of their completeness and the accuracy of recording. If you were to rely on these solely as a source of data you could experience problems.

Another consideration if you are relying on secondary sources is that you will be relying on someone else's interpretation of the data. You must be aware of this when using secondary sources of data. As you will see later, when we look at critical appraisal of research reports, one of the features that we should always look for in assessing research is the reliability of the information given.

It is because of the risks associated with relying on other people's sources of data that researchers are advised to use primary or direct sources of data wherever possible when undertaking research studies.

Direct sources of data

The techniques employed for collecting data directly can be grouped into two main categories:

- observation

- asking questions.

Within these categories the ways in which the data can be collected are varied. For example, observation studies can be undertaken by the researcher simply sitting and watching what is going on in a given situation – non-participant observation. Alternatively, the observer might choose to participate in some activities with the group being researched and undertake observations in the course of the activity – participant observation.

Researchers can ask questions directly by visiting a respondent at home or at work and undertaking face-to-face interviews. The data collected here are in a direct form because of the personal contact with the researcher.

Although asking questions can be a direct source of collecting data, the researcher doesn't always have direct contact with the person answering them. Most people today have had experience of questionnaires arriving in the post. In this situation the person responding to the questionnaire doesn't have direct contact with the researcher, but does respond directly to the researcher's questions. This is, therefore, indirect contact with the researcher.

Our two direct sources of data can therefore be broken down further, as shown in *Figure 4.1*.

Observation	● non-participant observation (direct data)
	● participant observation (direct data)
Asking questions	● questionnaire (direct or indirect contact with researcher)
	● interview (direct contact with researcher)

Figure 4.1: Types of direct data collection

List what you think would be the advantages of researchers collecting data directly themselves.

Commentary

The advantages of direct data collection are that:

1   Data collected directly from respondents are collected in the format the researcher requires.

2   Data coming straight from the respondents are perhaps more reliable than data derived from some secondary sources.

In the rest of this session we will consider in more detail how each of the following techniques of data collection can be used:

- observation
- asking questions by
  - questionnaires
  - interviews.

Observation

Observation is a very useful approach to research because it enables the researcher to observe first hand what is happening in a given situation and to see how people behave or respond to certain situations both physically and verbally. For example, we might want to undertake a study of how children behave when with their parents and when with other carers. By observing children in these two situations we could gather a lot of data that would otherwise not be available to us.

As noted above, a researcher can carry out non-participant observation by acting as an observer and simply watching what is happening. Alternatively, the researcher could work alongside the participants whilst observing the patterns of behaviour and carry out participant observation. A researcher who wanted to monitor the workload of a specific occupational group would need to be a non-participant observer, because if they became involved in doing the work of that group they would distort the picture they were trying to capture. However, in another situation a researcher could be a participant observer. If, for example, the researcher was a nurse studying the spread of infection in a hospital, she could work alongside other health workers and occasionally break off to observe particular practices.

The approach chosen obviously depends on the nature of the study. If a researcher is interested in examining how a particular cultural group responds to a given situation, it would not be appropriate to participate in those activities since such participation might influence the outcome of the research. A researcher might be interested in the way a team of health and social workers manage cases at a case conference (the meeting of the health care team and client in which client care is planned). If the researcher were an active participant in the conference it might change the group dynamic completely.

Alternatively, if a researcher is simply interested in one aspect of behaviour, it may be appropriate to help out in other aspects of the work and simply to stand back and observe when that particular aspect of behaviour is exhibited. If a researcher is interested in how social workers talk to elderly clients, he or she could be present at the case conference, so long as he or she kept quiet when the interaction he or she wished to observe was actually taking place.

ACTIVITY 41

ALLOW 5 MINUTES

1   List some instances related to your own area of practice where you think it could be useful to undertake a non-participant observational study.

2   What methods would you use to organise the information you gather as a result of your observations?

Commentary

1   You might have come up with ideas like:

● observing how your colleagues relate to patients or clients in certain situations

● observing how your patients or clients respond to treatments

● observing how particular groups behave in certain situations, for example, children in play school, teenagers' smoking habits, and so on.

2   There are a number of ways in which you can organise your observations and these will depend on the nature of the study you are undertaking. If you were undertaking a quantitative study you would need to use ways of gathering data that are amenable to quantification. For example, you might observe how often a professional has conversations with a client, who initiates the contact and how long each conversation lasts. You could also note the frequency of specified types of non-verbal communication. A simple check list such as that in *Figure 4.2* would give you a suitable

framework for gathering these data. This would be a highly structured observation schedule.

Alternatively, if you were undertaking a qualitative study and trying to understand a given situation, you might have a much more open observation sheet in which you simply noted events as they happened. *Figure 4.3* shows an example of this kind of low structure observation schedule.

COMMUNICATION RECORD

	Time contact took place; length of contact			
Verbal communication				
Client talks to social worker				
Social worker talks to client				
Non-verbal communication				
Social worker touches client				
Client smiles at social worker				

Figure 4.2: Example of an observation checklist for use in quantitative research

Meeting with social worker and client, 19 August 19XX

Comments on:

1) *Verbal communication*

2) *Non-verbal communication*

Figure 4 3: Example of an observation schedule for use in qualitative research

Observation – a research method in which a researcher observes subjects in order to gather data. Observation research comprises both 'participation' and 'non-participation' research methods. The participant observer observes the subjects from within by becoming a member of the group he or she is researching. The non-participant observer observes the subjects from without by observing the group as a researcher.

Managing observation studies

One of the major problems with observation studies is that they are a time-consuming means of data collection. Researchers need to consider the best way of collecting data within the time available – not only because of the time-consuming nature of observation design, but also because any observer who spends too long sitting in one place is likely to become tired themselves and this will influence the quality of his or her observations. To avoid problems in concentration two approaches are adopted in this type of study. These are 'time sampling' and 'event sampling'.

In time sampling, data are collected at fixed-time intervals on the assumption that the behaviour does not alter vastly over a certain time period. This method is very useful when wanting to capture activities over a long period of time. For example, a social worker may be interested in observing how elderly clients adapt to a new residential home. It would not be reasonable to spend a whole day observing what goes on in the home for two reasons: the first, concentration, and the second relating to the actual research question.

If a key area of concern was to see how new elderly clients interacted with other clients in the home there would be little value in observing clients at night when they are all, one assumes, asleep. The process of time sampling therefore involves selecting periods of time that would enable a researcher to gather relevant data without becoming exhausted. This might be in short slots of one hour throughout a day and would extend to as many hours as the researcher feels he or she can manage whilst keeping up his or her concentration.

Event sampling is used when a researcher wants to look at behavioural changes in circumstances which happen infrequently. For example, a nurse researcher may wish to observe how some aspects of care are carried out. Rather than spending periods of time generally observing, the researcher in this situation would only go and observe when an 'event' was actually occurring.

ACTIVITY 42 — ALLOW 10 MINUTES

1 What other difficulties do you think could arise when implementing an observation study?

2 Try to think of situations in your own practice in which it might be appropriate to use time or event sampling.

Commentary

1   One of the problems that you might have envisaged occurring could concern the person being observed. Subjects under observation could behave more favourably than usual and try to behave in the way they feel the observer wants them to behave. On the other hand, a participant might resent the fact that he or she is the subject of research and act accordingly. This pattern is well recognised in observation research and is commonly described as the 'Hawthorne effect' – after a study in an electrical plant in the USA where the phenomenon of altered behaviour in subjects being studied was first observed.

Another difficulty you may have thought of is that the observer might only see what he or she *wants* to see and dismiss any actions or responses that don't quite fit into his or her notions of what *should* be happening. People often reach conclusions using only a very limited amount of information and many of us have stereotypical ideas about certain groups of people which can greatly affect our judgement. We will go on to look at how one deals with these difficulties following the end of this commentary.

2   Any study that involves observing over a long period of time would be appropriate for time sampling. However, since it is not a good idea for researchers to spend long periods of time trying to concentrate, you could break your observations down into smaller time units totalling, for example, up to two hours throughout a 24-hour period.

You might choose to carry out event sampling if you were interested in watching how one specific procedure or task was performed, such as an interaction with a client or a specific nursing task or procedure. In these cases the researcher would arrange to be present when the event was occurring.

Reliability and validity of observations

As we have indicated above, there may be a number of reasons why observations may not be reliable. For example, we have suggested that a researcher may only see what he or she wants to see or that the people being observed may behave differently from normal when being observed.

In order to create a situation where people being observed are not affected by the presence of an observer, a researcher has to allow for a pre-observation period in which time is spent apparently observing, but not in fact doing so. This period of time is known as 'orientation time' – the researcher can refine the tool he or she intends to use in the study and the people being observed can get used to the presence of the observer. After a period of time people do become accustomed to researchers being present and thus the effects of observing can be reduced.

One-way screens or hidden video cameras can also be used so participants don't realise they are being watched and thus behave more naturally. However, this can cause ethical problems and so you would need to decide whether this observation technique was really essential. It would also, of course, be a more costly approach since such equipment can be expensive.

Observers frequently have their observations checked by an independent observer. If two people use the same observation schedule to record the same event, we can expect, if the observation schedule was reliable, that both would make the same observations. At the end of the observation period the two observers could compare notes to determine the level of reliability. This is known as 'interrater reliability'. One might think that having two observers would distort people's behaviour even further. However, experience indicates that this is not the case.

Indeed, once people have got used to an observer being present it does not even matter if this observer is later replaced by another.

In observation research we can say that validity is high since it is the only type of research where we report directly on what we see. However, as we noted above, researchers have to be very careful not to introduce bias into their observations by seeing only what they want to see.

ACTIVITY 43
ALLOW 60 MINUTES

The skills required to undertake observational research can take time to develop. You could begin to develop them when sitting alone in the following day-to-day situations.

1 Imagine that you are undertaking a qualitative study designed to look at how people behave in canteens. Using the one at work or college try simply observing what is happening around you. Make notes which will enable you to recall events later on.

2 On another occasion set yourself a quantitative observational task. Think about your average day at college or at work and consider the range of conversations that occur between individuals in that setting. Draw up a chart to monitor the frequency and length of each set of communications you observe.

3 Once you have completed 1 and 2 make notes about how easy or difficult you found each approach.

Commentary

You will find examples of both approaches below in *Figures 4.4* and *4.5* – read through them now. As you can see, the qualitative observation is written out in long-hand and consists of a series of observations relating to people collecting their food, eating food, interacting with colleagues and behaving in a tidy manner. If you tried to do this observation during a busy time you probably had difficulty writing everything down. Your notes would certainly not be as tidy as the script we have presented. What many observers would do in this situation would be to write very brief notes at the time and to write them up rather more neatly at a later stage (and this is actually what we did in this case.)

In the second example we have noted the range of time and frequency of occurrence of the events noted on our chart. We used a time-sampling procedure of one hour observing and one hour off. Again, you may not have found this easy to do.

The problem encountered with structured charts such as this is deciding whether what you are observing actually fits into one of your chosen categories.

For example, you may have noted that we have not recorded any communication between our manager and staff member of less that 30 seconds. What would we have done if the manager had made a passing comment to a staff member going in and out of the office? We would obviously have had to make a decision about whether or not to include this in our schedule. If you timed the communication sessions you were observing while you watched them you may have found it quite hard to make accurate records.

Each of these approaches to observation obviously has its strengths and weaknesses. Don't worry if you found this a hard exercise to do – the idea was simply to give you a feeling for the kind of problems researchers using observation techniques in data collection can face.

The canteen
Observation time 12.30 to 13.30

Comment

It is quite hard to keep up with the number of people collecting food – I see an endless stream of them going by. It is not possible to see what is on their plates, but I can see that the people concentrate a lot when choosing what to eat. There seem to be more men than women here today – I have only seen three women so far. Most other people using the canteen are my older colleagues – there is not much evidence of younger groups.

It is interesting to watch where people sit. A man in a brown jumper has gone to sit in the corner even though he has just talked to the man in the black suit at another table. Most people seem to be eating in a hurry – they are getting their meals, hurrying them down and rushing away. The man in the brown jumper was in and out in ten minutes.

People are very tidy – they nearly all moved their trays out of the way.

Figure 4.4: Example of completed observation schedule (qualitative data)

Communication record **Verbal communication**	time 9-10am	time 11-12md	time 1-2pm	time 3-4pm	time 5-6pm
Manager talks to staff member	5 mins	30secs	1 min	5 mins	
Staff member talks to manager	30 secs	3 mins	1 min		
Non-verbal communication (frequency noted by X)					
Manager looks at staff member	X X XX	X	X	-	-
Staff member touches client	X	XXX	XX	X	X

Figure 4.5: Example of completed observation checklist (quantitative data)

Asking questions

The other means of collecting data is actually to ask subjects questions – either through the use of self-completed questionnaires or by interviewing them.

Questionnaires

Questionnaire – a tool for data collection in research. May be highly structured and contain only **closed questions** or have low structure and contain many **open questions**. It is not unusual for questionnaires to have a mix of both open and closed questions.

Questionnaires are a very popular means of eliciting information and they have many advantages over other techniques. Most people have had some experience of completing questionnaires and this might be a reason why they are so popular with researchers.

In order to look at the advantages and disadvantages of questionnaires consider the following case study.

Jenny and **Jo** work together in a health care centre. They have decided that they would like to carry out a study to identify the factors that influence whether people use the health promotion unit in the clinic. They have a debate about how best to do this. Jenny feels that it might be a good idea to observe people who visit the unit and see how they make use of the resources, but Jo feels that this will only focus on those people actually using the unit and it will not help to find out why other people do not use the unit. After some discussion they decide that the best way forward would be to prepare a questionnaire to send to a sample of clients registered with the health centre.

Both Jenny and Jo are aware of the pros and cons of using questionnaires. They made their decision knowing that the advantages of questionnaires are that they:

- are relatively inexpensive

- provide large batches of data which can be handled in a quick and efficient way

- provide findings which are easy to analyse

- provide replies which, being anonymous, are more likely to be honest – particularly if the questions are of a personal or sensitive nature.

Jenny and Jo chose to use a questionnaire even though they know that it can have the following drawbacks:

- it is quite difficult to design a good questionnaire

- respondents often have a fixed-choice of answers so that the answers they give may not be a true representation of what they really think or feel

- because there is no contact between the person asking the questions and the participant, any ambiguities in the questions cannot be clarified

- the return rate of questionnaires is generally quite low.

Designing questionnaires

The approach you decide to use in your research will obviously have an impact on the design of your questionnaires. Questionnaires for use in quantitative studies involve the use of some form of measurement which assigns numerical values to each of the different responses to the questions. Using questionnaires in qualitative research involves asking more open questions, to which the respondents reply in their own words.

Taking advantage of the benefits of questionnaires

We will now consider how to use the known advantages of questionnaires to help in planning a study that might involve their use.

1 *Questionnaires are relatively inexpensive*

The time taken to print and circulate a hundred questionnaires is much less than the comparable time taken to interview a hundred people or to observe a hundred episodes of care. However, one mustn't underestimate the amount of time it can take to develop a good, reliable questionnaire (reliability referring to the degree of consistency with which a research instrument measures what it is supposed to measure).

2 *Large batches of data can be handled in a quick and efficient way*

This advantage will depend on the degree of care you give to designing your questionnaire. As you will recall, questions can have a high or low structure and obviously the more structured the questions and responses, the clearer the data they will yield.

3 *The findings from questionnaires are easy to analyse*

If questions have high structure (i.e. the respondents have only a limited range of choices when responding to each question) data can be handled quickly and efficiently provided sufficient thought is given at the outset to how this will be done.

A very common problem faced by newcomers to research is that they find they have failed to think about what they will do with the data when they analyse it and so this apparent advantage does not materialise. For example, if a researcher had asked someone to answer a question that had more than one response, such as selecting several factors one enjoys about work, they would find this more difficult to analyse than a simple 'yes/no' question. It is harder to decide what to do with data once you have got them than to plan what you will do beforehand. Failure to do this can also result in wasted data.

4 *Since data can be gathered anonymously, the replies are more likely to be honest – particularly if the questions are of a personal or sensitive nature*

This point can be quite important when researching a sensitive area. People will often only cooperate with research into sensitive topics if they know that they can remain anonymous. It is also very important that researchers carrying out questionnaires which aren't anonymous assure potential respondents that the data will be handled in confidence.

Sidestepping the disadvantages of questionnaires

Here we will consider how to avoid the pitfalls associated with questionnaires.

It is actually quite difficult to design a good questionnaire.
Several textbooks have been written on questionnaire design (see, for example, Oppenheim ,1992) and so it is unrealistic to try and address that issue in full here! However, some practical tips about general layout that are worth considering at this stage are:

Clear instructions

You should make it very clear to respondents exactly what you want them to do. Ambiguous instructions can result in ambiguous responses. Do not worry about spelling out your orders – if you want respondents to tick a box then say so ('Tick the box that applies to you').

Keep it simple

It is always helpful to put yourself in the place of the person you are expecting to respond to your questionnaire. If you were asked to help out in a research study by completing a questionnaire you might be quite happy to spend a few minutes filling out a form, but you would not be so happy if the form took a couple of hours of your time.

- Place the questions in a *logical sequence* to make it easier for respondents to fully comprehend the meaning of a question.

- As well as looking at the order of the questions, you will need to spend a great deal of time on the actual *phrasing* of the questions. The following tips should be remembered.

- Always use *simple language*, i.e. one syllable words instead of three syllable words. It is far better to say 'did you travel by bus?' than to ask 'did you travel by road-based public transport systems?'.

- Be specific in order to *avoid ambiguity*. You should avoid using words like 'frequently' or 'regularly' since people have their own interpretation of what these terms mean.

- Avoid *leading questions* such as 'don't you think that..?' and 'isn't it true that...?'. These can greatly influence peoples' responses and can cause them not to be totally honest and thus to create unreliable data!

- Only ask *one thing at a time* – avoid using words like 'and' and 'or' in a question. For example, it is better to say 'do you take sugar in your tea?' than to ask 'do you take milk and sugar in your tea?'. The latter question could not be responded to with a simple 'yes' or 'no'.

Respondents often have a fixed-choice of answers. Consequently, the answers they give may not be a true representation of what they really think or feel

People making a case for qualitative research often criticise the high structure of quantitative questionnaires. However, although these responses are fixed-choice, the researchers who develop the rating scales used to analyse the responses do make efforts to ensure that these scales are reliable and valid.

There are many, well-established scale techniques which are very popular and easy to implement. Basically, they involve assigning to 'traits' or 'statements' a numerical figure on a scale. Examples of these can be seen in *Figure 4.6*.

Evaluation scales are where 'marks out of 5' are awarded, e.g.

On the scale below where 1 = highest and 5 = lowest , indicate how much you enjoy your job

1 ☐☐☐☐☐ 5

Comparative scales are where two or more aspects are ranked in order of importance, e.g.

The following list indicates features of your job that you may enjoy. Indicate in order of priority what is most important to you using 1 = most important and 5 = least important

working relationships with colleagues	☐
light airy office	☐
good administrative support	☐
supportive manager	☐
interesting work	☐

Attitude scales are where subjects state how they feel about certain statements by using numerical values. One of the most common attitude scales is the 'Likert scale' in which people are asked to agree or disagree with statements relating to the area of study. So, for example, if a researcher was trying to find out what people thought about using research in their practice, a section from a Likert scale would look like this:

Statement	SA	A	U	D	SD	Total
I feel confident that I can tell the difference between a poor and an adequate research report						
I am confident that my practice is based on the most recent research findings						
I have not received sufficient education to be able to understand a research report						

SA = Strongly Agree A = Agree U = Undecided D = Disagree SD = Strongly Disagree

Figure 4.6: Examples of rating scales

Although it is helpful for newcomers to research to learn about well-established measurement scales, you should note that many of these are subject to copyright by the people who developed them. If you wanted to use such scales in a research study you would need to get permission. Permission may be granted for some scales, but for others you might be required to show evidence that you have the necessary knowledge and skills to use them. This means that in practice not all established scales are available for use by all researchers.

Since there is no contact between the person asking the questions and the participant, any ambiguities in the questions cannot be clarified

It is possible to deal with this at the design stage. If a researcher develops a questionnaire that is reliable and valid it should not have many ambiguities by the time it reaches the target group.

The actual return rate of questionnaires tends to be quite low

Response rates to questionnaires can be improved in a number of ways – for instance, by providing the participants with stamped addressed envelopes (although this will obviously make the process much more costly). Reminder letters can also help.

ACTIVITY 44 ALLOW 15 MINUTES

Read the case study in the box below and suggest the kinds of points Janie's supervisor might make about:

a) What is good in the questionnaire.

b) What is poor in the questionnaire.

Janie works as a fitness instructor in a health centre. She has a theory that people who attend the centre, who take exercise regularly and who also do not smoke feel happier than those who do not take exercise and who smoke more than 20 cigarettes a day. Janie decides to conduct some research on this topic as she is taking a course of study which requires her to carry out a research paper of some kind.

She recognises that to give a questionnaire to people who attend the local centre would introduce bias because these people obviously take exercise regularly, so she decides to administer her questionnaire to a group of people attending a local summer fair . She gets permission from the organisers to circulate her questionnaire as people arrive (see questionnaire in *Figure 4.7*).

> When Janie goes to see her course supervisor Hilary, with the first draft of her questionnaire, the supervisor has a lot of comments to make about it – some positive and some negative.

Draft 1
Health Questionnaire

1. Do you smoke frequently?

2. Don't you think that exercise is good for you if you have time?

3. How old are you?

4. Isn't it true that it is better not to smoke?

5. Do you take exercise regularly?

6. Isn't it true that you feel happy most of the time?

7. Don't you feel that we should all diet and take exercise?

Figure 4.7: Janie's first draft of her questionnaire

Commentary

1 Hilary, Janie's supervisor, is unlikely to find very much that is good in this questionnaire! One of the few points in its favour is its brevity – it won't be too daunting to anyone seeing it for the first time. One could also cite question 5 as an example of a straightforward question.

2 This questionnaire makes all the mistakes we noted above in our list of problems with questionnaire design:

- there are no clear instructions as to what the respondents are supposed to do

- ambiguous words and phrases are included in the questions – words such as 'frequently' or 'regularly' mean different things to different people

- it uses leading questions such as 'don't you think that...' and 'don't you feel...'

- it asks respondents to say how old they are – some people are sensitive about this and so it is better to indicate an age range

- there is no logical sequence to the questions asked.

Obviously Hilary is going to have to give Janie some advice! What happens next is described in the box below.

Hilary gives Janie some practical tips about following the format identified in an introductory research text. Janie goes away to develop a second draft of her questionnaire (see *Figure 4.8*).

Looking at the second draft, Hilary can immediately see that it is a rather better format. She thinks it would be possible to look at the data produced in this questionnaire and use it to identify whether people in certain age and gender groups believe in the value of exercise, how many of them smoke and how many of them are happy. Hilary also suggests that it would be possible to look at those who feel happy and compare this with their views on exercise.

Hilary now suggests that Janie undertakes a pilot study with the questionnaire.

The questionnaire in *Figure 4.8* is set out in a much more logical form than that in *Figure 4.7*. The instructions are clear and the questions are more focused. Janie has taken the ambiguous words and phrases out of her questions. However, she cannot claim that it is a reliable and valid questionnaire until she has undertaken a pilot study to test the questionnaire. Still, for a second draft of a questionnaire it looks quite promising. You can now help to test this questionnaire.

Draft 2

Health Questionnaire

Please tick the appropriate response

1. Please indicate your age: 15-20 ☐ 21-30 ☐ 31-40 ☐ 41-50 ☐

2. Please indicate whether you are: male ☐ female ☐

3. Do you take exercise regularly? Yes ☐ No ☐

4. Do you take time each day to exercise? Yes ☐ No ☐

4.1. If your answer to question 4 is 'yes' please indicate how long you exercise for each day:

   10 minutes ☐ 20 minutes ☐ 30 minutes ☐ more than 30 minutes ☐

5. Do you smoke? Yes ☐ No ☐

5.1 If your answer to question 5 is 'yes' please indicate how many cigarettes each day:
   1-5 ☐ 6-10 ☐ 11-15 ☐ 16-20 ☐ 21-25 ☐ more than 25 ☐

6. Please indicate which of the following statements describes how you feel:

   I feel happy most of the time ☐

   I feel happy some of the time ☐

   I never feel happy. ☐

Figure 4.8: Janie's second draft of her questionnaire

ACTIVITY 45

1 Make ten copies of the questionnaire in *Figure 4.8*. (Photocopy the original if you can or type it out again if you have access to a word processor. Do not handwrite it as this can adversely affect the overall presentation and may influence the way in which people respond.)

2 Ask ten of your colleagues or friends to complete the questionnaire for you in your presence and asking for clarification where necessary.

3 Take note of:

● how long it takes each person to complete it

● whether your respondents need you to clarify any of the questions (if yes which ones)

● whether they objected to any of the questions (if yes, which ones).

4 Collate the responses to each question. To do this use a blank questionnaire and record on it how many people have responded to each choice available. For example, if six respondents say 'yes' to question 4 and four say 'no', then write six in the 'yes' box and four in the 'no' box.

Commentary

Did this exercise reveal any problems with the questionnaire? Which questions were noted as being difficult to answer or objectionable?

Hang on to these completed questionnaires, as we will be returning to them later on.

Interview techniques

The word 'interview' usually describes a situation where a researcher asks a participant face-to-face questions. There are many advantages to collecting information in this way:

● depending on the length of the interview, results can be obtained very quickly

● the person being interviewed has the opportunity to ask for clarification if he or she does not understand exactly what is being asked of them

● the interviewer can also ask for clarification if responses are not precise enough.

Interviews can either be 'unstructured' or 'structured'. In a 'structured interview' the researcher decides beforehand what questions to ask and uses a structured questionnaire to focus on these questions. In an unstructured interview the interviewee is asked to speak about a certain topic with 'prompts' and questions from the researcher as the need arises. This would be the approach adopted in a qualitative design study.

For example, a researcher interviewing staff in a health centre might ask 'Please tell me your views about the Community Care Act.' If taking an unstructured approach, the interviewer may not want to ask any further formal questions, but he or she might have some idea of the areas he or she would like covered in the responses. For example, he or she might want to be sure that each interviewee made some comment on the impact of the Community Care Act on working relationships with colleagues and clients. In order to ensure that such comments were made, the interviewer might need to prompt interviewees for their views on this.

Another advantage of interviews is their response rate. Janie used a written questionnaire but she could have decided to collect her data by interviewing people using the questionnaire format. This way she would probably get a higher response rate than if she asked people to complete it themselves.

Although interviews do have advantages, they can also cause problems that don't arise when using questionnaires. It is possible, for example, that when actually faced with an interviewer a respondent may give the answers he or she believes the interviewer wants to hear. In highly structured interviews, such as Janie's second draft questionnaire above, the researcher must always ask the questions in the same way. This is made easier if the questions are well phrased.

A 'semi structured' or 'focused' interview may give researchers more scope for asking questions and probing, but they need to be particularly aware of the problem of influence. Inexperienced researchers often lack the skill to probe without influencing responses.

ACTIVITY 46 — ALLOW 60 MINUTES

For this exercise you need to find four or five colleagues to help you.

Ask each person the following questions:

- what are your views on taking exercise?

- what are your views on smoking?

Make notes of the responses you get and then consider the following issues:

- was it easy to get a response?

- what problems did you encounter in trying to get a response?

Commentary

The kind of problems interviewers commonly encounter in getting people to respond to open questions include:

- getting interviewees sufficiently relaxed to respond

- distractions from other sources while interviews are underway

- interviewees digressing from the actual question asked.

Another kind of problem interviewers encounter is keeping notes of what is going on. We asked you to note down what people said so that you might experience this problem. It is, of course, much easier for interviewers to use a tape recorder to note responses, but this can create problems as sometimes people are more sensitive about being recorded than they would be about simply answering the question.

In this session you have had the opportunity to undertake observations, ask colleagues to complete a short questionnaire and carry out some interviews. By this stage you should be beginning to understand each approach in terms of the kind of data that you can collect and the way in which you can collect them.

We will now look at the differences between the data you collected from your questionnaires and the data you collected in the interviews.

ACTIVITY 47 — ALLOW 5 MINUTES

Consider the data collected from the interviews and the questionnaire. What do you see as the main differences between the two sets of data?

Commentary

In the questionnaire you asked people very specific questions and got quite specific responses. You can count these responses and indicate the results in numerical form.

The semi-structured interviews will have produced data that cannot be measured so easily because your interviewees' views on exercise and smoking are probably quite varied.

This demonstrates the fundamental design difference between the two approaches. In the structured questionnaire we used deductive reasoning to design the questionnaire – that is, we used some existing knowledge to help us define frequency of exercise, smoking patterns and so on. This is a quantitative approach in which we can count the number of responses to each section.

In the interviews we started with two general topics but asked the interviewees to tell us what they thought. Here we used an inductive approach because we hoped that ideas would be generated by the topics. This is a qualitative approach in which the data will be analysed in words. This is in contrast to the structured questionnaire used earlier, in which we talked about collating the number of responses. Here the data are managed in written format and rather than counting responses we will be looking for the meaning in words (sentences and statements.)

Pilot studies

A pilot study is a small-scale version of a study. It is carried out before the real study takes place.

It creates the opportunity for you to test the tools you have designed to see whether they work. Once you have finished constructing a questionnaire or interview schedule it is always advisable to undertake a pilot study to ensure that there are no fundamental problems with the design. For example, have people had problems answering questions which were ambiguous? Was the fact that you required the subject to tick only one box not clear enough? And so on. Although this may seem a tedious process, piloting research tools can save an immense amount of time and money in the long run. If your research tools are poor then your research will be poor.

You have already participated in two exercises that could be classed as pilot studies:

- by asking your colleagues to complete a draft questionnaire and

- by undertaking short interviews.

If you encountered any problems while conducting those exercises you will perhaps already appreciate the value of a pilot study.

Once you have completed your pilot study you can make amendments to your research tool as necessary. When you later proceed with the study you can do so knowing that your techniques or methods of data collection will actually work for you.

Summary

In Session Four we have discussed issues fundamental to research design:

1 Reliability of research instruments to give results that are consistent.

2 Validity of research instruments to measure what is intended.

3 Gathering data from direct and indirect sources.

4 Recognising how bias can be introduced into research design.

Before you move on to Session Five check that you have achieved the objectives given at the beginning of this session and, if not, review the appropriate sections.

SESSION FIVE

Data analysis

Introduction

The purpose of this session is to give you a very basic introduction to the ways in which data collected in both quantitative and qualitative research studies are analysed. We will begin by looking at quantitative data analysis and considering some of the principles of descriptive and inferential statistics. We will then explore content analysis in qualitative research.

Session objectives

When you have completed this session you should be able to:

- explain the purpose of using statistics in data analysis

- state what is meant by the terms: the mean, the range, the median, the mode and the standard deviation

- contrast descriptive statistics with inferential statistics

- outline what is meant by 'a risk of error' in an inferential statistics test

- describe the first step in qualitative data analysis.

1: Principles of data analysis

The approach a researcher uses for data analysis depends entirely on his or her overall research design. This is because the analysis of data depends on how those data were collected. It is vitally important to remember that the means for analysing the data should be decided at the research design stage, ie. *before* the data have been gathered. It is not uncommon for new researchers to plan a study, design their tools for data collection, collect the data and only then question what they will actually do with the data once they have got them!

Analysing information

We looked briefly at a form of statistical analysis in Session Three when we presented data indicating the frequency with which elderly patients visited the GP (see *Table 5.1* below). We noted that the data were presented using 'descriptive statistics' – which simply means *describing* the occurrence of visits to the GP in *numerical form*. Statistics are simply a way of summarising data.

In this example we presented our information in numerical form, indicating the actual number of visits. To support this, we used percentage ratings to give some further meaning to the figures cited. If we had just said that the number of patients visiting the surgery in January was 50 this would not have been very meaningful; however, if we say that the number of patients visiting the surgery in January was 50 and that this represents 10 per cent of the total visits by the elderly to the GP for the year, the information starts to become more meaningful.

Similarly, if we had said that 10 per cent of the visits were undertaken in January without giving some indication of the actual numbers of patients involved this might also prove to be inadequate information. If the total attendance for the year of this client group had only been 20 then 10 per cent would represent only two people visiting the surgery. This is useful to know as in health and social research it is common for the results of small research studies to be published. When reading such reports you always need to check the actual numbers involved, as this will influence the reliability of the study. So, remember an important thing to look out for in research reports is *what the numbers in the data actually represent.*

Month	Number of cases visiting the doctor	
January	50	(10%)
February	70	(14%)
March	55	(12%)
April	50	(10%)
May	45	(9%)
June	35	(7%)
July	25	(5%)
August	15	(3%)
September	30	(6%)
October	25	(5%)
November	45	(9%)
December	45	(9%)
Total	500	(100%)

Key: percentages represent the percentage of total visits by elderly people to the doctor during the year.

Table 5.1: Number of elderly people visiting the GP surgery (repeated from Session Three)

ACTIVITY 48   ALLOW **10** MINUTES

1 Turn again to *Resource 1* and note the way Rita Howard reported the results for older people attending the A & E department.

2 What might Howard's reasons have been for choosing to provide her data in the form she did, rather than using a table?

Commentary

1 In this paper Howard has used a chart to illustrate the range of reasons why people attended the A & E department and has then discussed the actual ratings in the text itself.

2 If Howard had presented her data in a table showing figures and percentages she couldn't have provided such a clear presentation of the total attendances against the justified attendances. However there are no 'rights and wrongs' in this situation. Each researcher will choose what he or she considers to be the most comprehensive way of presenting his or her data.

2: Data analysis in quantitative designs

The basic premise of data analysis in quantitative design is that the data will be subject to some form of calculation. The level of calculation required will vary, from a simple description of the frequency with which a particular response occurs, to a more complex analysis in which this frequency is compared with other sources of data.

This way of presenting data offers a useful summary that can save a great deal of time in long-winded description. You can present in one line of figures a lot of data that would take many lines of words to explain. The figures that are used most frequently are those called the 'mean' and the 'range'. You also need to know about those called the 'median' and 'mode' for when we look at some of the more complex ways of using statistics in health and social care research later on. In the example of attendance at the GP's surgery above, we have simply calculated the frequency of visits.

The mean

Mean – *A measure used in descriptive statistics to identify the average score in a set of figures. It provides a means of summarising data and gives an indication of the central tendency of a set of figures.*

If we take the information (data) about the GP's surgery and look at it more closely we can identify a number of features in it. For example, if we look at the total attendance for the year, we note that there were 500 visits to the GP. If we then divide that by the 12 months of the year we can say that the *average attendance* per month over the year is 41.6 patients per month. In statistical terms the average is referred to as the '**mean**'.

In most situations it is useful to know the mean. For example, the mean of 41.6 noted in the GP's surgery could differ from the mean attendance of only 30 elderly people at another surgery. This would affect how those planning health and social care allocated resources to support service provision. They might feel that a surgery with a lower attendance rate does not need as many resources as one with a higher rate.

The mean is, however, only one measure and giving the overall average would not in itself give a clear indication of workload on a month-by-month basis. We can see from *Table 5.1* that the 'range' of visits – that is, the lowest number and the highest number – to the GP's surgery varies from 15 visits in August to 70 visits in February. This has implications for the allocation of resources in those particular months. It might, for example, be preferable for the health and social care staff to plan their holidays in the month of August rather than in February when peak attendance may be anticipated.

Two other sets of figures are sometimes referred to in describing the distribution of a set of results. The first of these is the 'median', which is the mid-point figure. The second is the 'mode', which indicates the most frequently occurring figure.

The median

If we look at the statistics from *Table 5.1* and set out the frequency of visits in numerical order the figures look like this:

15   25   25   30   35   45   45   45   50   50   55   70

Median – *a measure used in descriptive statistics to indicate central tendency in a set of figures by identifying the score which falls exactly in the middle of a set of figures.*

The figure that sits exactly in the mid-point of this data is 45 and this is the **median**. The median is a descriptive statistic that is a measure of 'central tendency'. It is the figure that is the central point of a set of observations. This is important for some statistical tests, as researchers may be required to identify the median under calculatory formulae. It is not used as frequently as the mean and you should note that there can be a difference between the mean score and the median score. For example, in our calculation of the mean above we noted that for this set of data the mean is 41.6. This figure is quite close to the median. Now, however, look at another a set of figures in (a):

(a)   2   3   4   10   16.

The mean for this set of scores is 7, yet the median (the central figure) is only 4. We do not know how many numbers are placed below the median or how many there are above. The median would still be four if we added three more sets of data to our figures – see (b) where the mean is 30.3.

(b) 1   2   2   2   2   4   10   16   98   98   99

To calculate the median where there are an even number of figures, you need to add the two middle figures together and then find the mean of these two. Thus, if we had to calculate the median for (c), for example, we would add 8 and 10 together and then divide by 2, giving a median of 9.

(c)   5   7   8   10   11   12

The mode

In the figures in *Table 5.1* you will see that the most frequently occurring number is 45. This number is known as the '**mode**' and again this is quite similar to the mean (41.6).

In examples (a) to (c) above, only one set of data (b) has a figure that occurs more than once, i.e. 2. For (b) we have already noted that the median is 4 and that the mean is 30.3. Here there is little similarity between the median, the mean and the mode, so you can see that sometimes the median, mean and mode are similar, and sometimes they are not.

As we have noted above, it is important for you to know the difference between the mean, median and mode. Some statistical tests that you will learn about later in your research course will demand this basic knowledge of descriptive statistics.

Mode – a measure used in descriptive statistics to describe the most frequently occurring number in a set of figures. This is a measure of central tendency.

ACTIVITY 49	ALLOW 10 MINUTES

Look at the set of figures from a second GP's surgery in *Table 5.2* and work out the answers to the following questions.

1 What is the total number of patients visiting this surgery over the year? Write out these figures as a set.

2 What is the range?

3 What is the mean?

4 What is the median?

5 What is the mode?

Month	Number of cases visiting the doctor
January	15
February	78
March	45
April	23
May	67
June	10
July	5
August	89
September	34
October	13
November	21
December	60
Total	460
Key: The figures represent the total number of people who visited the surgery in each month	

Table 5.2: Number of elderly people visiting a second GP's surgery

Commentary

1   The total number of patients attending the surgery in this year is 460. The set of figures is:

    5   10   13   15   21   23   34   45   60   67   78   89

2   The range is 5 to 89.

3   The mean is 38.3 (i.e. 460 /12).

4   In this set of figures we have two numbers at the mid-point – 23 and 34. To calculate the median we need to add these two together, then find the average and use that as the median, i.e. (23 + 34)/2 = 28.5.

5   There is not a mode in this set of figures as no number occurs more than once.

There is one more measure of central tendency that it is useful to know about and that is the standard deviation (SD). This is an important measure as it tells us how far a set of scores varies from the mean score. The greater the range, or 'dispersion', in a set of figures, the greater the numerical value of the standard deviation. If we read that the standard deviation of two sets of scores is as follows:

$$SD = 1.2$$

$$SD = 3.6$$

we know that there was a greater range in the figures used to calculate the SD in the second than in the first. It is useful to know about this test, as it is commonly used in health and social research as a means of summarising information.

The full formula for calculating the SD can be found in Miller (1994) in this series. Please refer to this if you want to find out more about the formula.

These five factors (the range, the median, the mean, the mode and the standard deviation) are all forms of 'descriptive statistics' – that is, they simply describe the data as seen - as opposed to analysing it in detail.

Another type of statistical analysis is known as 'inferential statistics'. For the moment we will simply introduce you to the notion of inferential statistical testing and the way in which the results from these types of statistics are presented.

As indicated by its name, this approach to statistics involves an attempt to *infer* something from the data. In other words, inferential statistics offer us a way of being able to *generalise* our findings from a smaller sample to the population as a whole. When using inferential statistics we are moving beyond the kind of descriptive data that we have outlined above.

The simple reason why we need inferential statistics is that they help us to discover whether our findings in any research study are due simply to chance or whether they are in fact likely to be correct. We will now illustrate this using a short case study.

Phyllis is a practice nurse working in a GP's surgery. She has noticed that some patients attending the practice have frequent urinary tract infections. As she reads the notes about these patients she begins to realise that those with the highest rate of infections appear to have a lower daily fluid intake than those with the lower rate of infections.

She proposes a simple hypothesis that states 'people with a low daily fluid intake are more likely to have urinary tract infections than those with a high fluid intake'. In this case she is proposing a relationship between the level of fluid intake (independent variable) and the incidence of urinary tract infection (dependent variable).

Phyllis could collect information relating to her patients, calculate the frequency of occurrence of urinary tract infections over the year and match this alongside the average daily intake of fluids in litres of a sample of her patients. These data are shown in *Table 5.3*.

Daily intake of fluids (in litres)	Number of urinary tract infections in year
1	3
1.5	3
2	2
2.5	2
2.5	1
3	1
3.5	0

Table 5.3: Daily intake of fluid against number of urinary tract infections over one year

ACTIVITY 50

Look at the small set of results Phyllis has gathered. Can you draw any conclusions from the data?

Commentary

The people who take the most fluids daily appear to have a lower incidence of urinary tract infections. If this pattern was reflected in all the patients attending the surgery we might feel that there is an association between the two factors and that a low fluid intake is somehow related to urinary tract infections.

By looking at these data Phyllis could calculate some descriptive statistics and note, for example, the mean fluid intake and the mean level for urinary tract infections. However, this will not tell her much more than she can see already. What she wants to know is whether she can *infer* something from these data. Is there is a significant relationship between fluid intake and urinary tract infection? The pattern identified could just be due to chance. In order to determine whether the pattern is due to *more than* chance, Phyllis would have to undertake an inferential statistical test.

Inferential statistical tests involve selecting a random sample from a population to test a particular hypothesis or statement and, using the results of that sample, making a conclusion about the population as a whole. In our example Phyllis has stated a hypothesis that *'people with a lower daily fluid intake are more likely to have urinary tract infections than those with a high fluid intake'*.

Inferential tests are known as 'tests of significance' – that is, they seek to detect 'significant' effects as distinct from chance effects. What Phyllis wants to know is whether what she is observing is significant or whether it is just a chance pattern.

Although tests of significance help to give a clear indication, they can never be taken as absolutely correct – there is always the possibility of error. The level of error that we might see as acceptable depends on the nature of the topic being studied. For example, where a researcher is undertaking a study that involves a new drug any degree of error might impact on many lives.

In most health and social research there is a general acceptance that a reasonable probability or degree of certainty that a conclusion is wrong is 5 per 100, that is 5 per cent. This means that if what is called the 'probability of error' in a study was calculated as being higher than 5 per cent the conclusion of the study would be less reliable than if the probability of error was 5 per cent or lower. All statistical tests in inferential statistics will produce conclusions based on stated probabilities of error. The results are usually written in decimal format. So a conclusion for a statistical test which had a 5 per cent risk of error would be written as '**P=.05**', **P** being probability. If the final calculation in a statistical test is less than 5 per cent the symbol '<' is used. If the final calculation is greater than 5 per cent the symbol ' >' is used. Thus, a result could be written as:

P < .05 (probability is less than 5 per cent – this is significant)

P > .05 (probability is more that 5 per cent – this is not significant).

If we refer back to the study that Phyllis is undertaking, she might find that as a result of her statistical tests the probability was P=.05. In this case she would be able to infer that there *was* a significant relationship between the level of fluid intake and the number of urinary tract infections over the year. She could state that her hypothesis *'people with a lower daily fluid intake are more likely to have urinary infections'* is supported.

ACTIVITY 51 — ALLOW 5 MINUTES

Assuming a level of significance of P=.05, look at the following P values and write down which ones you think might be significant.

1 P > .07

2 P < .04

3 P > .09

4 P < .01

5 P < .03

Commentary

You should have noted the following:

1 P > .07 : this is not significant as it is more than P=.05 at 7 per cent (i.e. 7 in 100)

2 P < .04 : this is significant as it is less than P=.05 at 4 per cent (i.e. 4 in 100)

3 P > .09 : this is not significant as this is more than P=.05 at 9 per cent (i.e. 9 in 100)

4 P < .01 : this is significant as this is less than P=.05 at 1 per cent (i.e. 1 in 100)

5 P < .03 : this is significant as this is less than P=.05 at 3 per cent (i.e. 3 in 100)

There is a wide range of inferential statistical tests but we will not be exploring these in this text. Our purpose here is simply to introduce you to the ideas of statistical testing and to help you to recognise some of the terms and abbreviations that are used in statistics. We will be returning to statistical testing in other units in this series. There is a range of textbook titles about statistics included in the Further Reading section to help you if you wish to explore further at this stage.

3: Data analysis in qualitative designs

The approach to data analysis in qualitative research is different to that used in quantitative analysis. As you will recall, qualitative research involves looking for meaning in words rather than figures.

ACTIVITY 52   ALLOW 15 MINUTES

Turn back to the article in *Resource 2* and remind yourself how the authors presented their data. How does this differ from the way in which the data were presented in the Howard article in *Resource 1*?

Commentary

The style of presentation in the two articles is quite different. Whilst Howard presents her data in a chart and with ratings in the text, Finn and Norman present their findings in themes, focusing on general issues identified in their research. They don't present their data in any numerical way. The authors state that they have taken this view because other sources of information have not generated the kind of information they need to study their chosen topic.

Qualitative data analysis is quite a time-consuming process and demands a lot of effort by the researcher. This may be a reason why it is not often used by new researchers. We will only provide a simple description of it at this stage, because the process will be considered in more detail in Unit 2 of this series.

Look back at the interviews you had with your colleagues in the Session Four activity about exercise and smoking. How do you think you would begin trying to analyse these data?

First of all, you would need to have the interview written out in full or 'transcribed'. Then you would need to look for common patterns in the responses. There are two ways you could do this:

1   You could make a more detailed breakdown of all the words in the data, looking at how frequently particular words or phrases recur.

2   You could try to identify general themes. We can look at this more closely in the following case study.

> **Teresa** has undertaken some interviews with mothers, asking their views of a new system for organising child care in the community. An extract from one of her interviews follows:
>
> 'I don't think it is a very good system, I mean it works quite well perhaps if you have only got one child, but it doesn't really help me with my three children. Organising them all is a major task. No sooner do I drop the oldest off than I have to go and collect the next one – it seems as if I am on the road all day. There must be a better way of organising this so that we can co-ordinate the care of all the children regardless of age.'

Although this is only a small piece of data we can state several things about it. The first is that all the data are in words! (In contrast to the data presented in *Tables 5.1 and 5.2*.) We can see a number of ideas in the data such as:

● number of children

● organising them all

● on the road

● co-ordinating care.

In this short piece we get the impression of a busy mother rushing around every day trying to co-ordinate care for her children. As Teresa is undertaking a number of interviews, what she will be looking for is to see whether any similar patterns emerge in the other data she collects.

ACTIVITY 53   ALLOW 30 MINUTES

Look back at your own interview data from the interview you carried out with colleagues about exercise and smoking. See if any patterns are evident in it. Concentrate for now on the views your respondents expressed about exercise. Are there any trends emerging in the data you have collected – common words or issues that keep appearing?

Commentary

> You may have found that the people you interviewed gave similar responses to your questions about exercise or you may have found some quite conflicting views. What you should be able to do at this stage is simply to summarise what you have found. Once you have done this simple activity you have taken the first step in qualitative data analysis. The techniques required for more in-depth analysis of qualitative data are explored further in the companion unit *Qualitative Methodology* (Clifford, 1996).

4: Some final thoughts on analysis

You will recall that in Session Four we explored the concepts of reliability, validity and bias. Before we move on from this section on data analysis you need to know that we are concerned with these issues at *all stages* of the research process. In the analysis stage we must take care not to undermine the reliability of our results by undertaking inappropriate statistical tests. We must also be careful not to misinterpret the data we are presented with in qualitative design. To help us do this there are quite stringent guidelines available to guide us through our process of data analysis in both quantitative and qualitative research. We have introduced you to some general principles of analysis here and direct you to the Further Reading section for a list of books which will give you a more in-depth review of the process of data analysis.

Summary

1   In Session Five you were introduced to a range of data analysis techniques in:

    a) quantitative research design

    b) qualitative research design

2   Using the information gained from this session you should be in a position to move on to Session Six.

Before moving on to Session Six check that you have achieved the objectives given at the beginning of this session, and, if not, review the appropriate sections.

SESSION SIX

Review

Introduction

In this last session we are going to explore the areas you need to consider when reading research reports and assessing the overall quality of the research reported. We will then help you to evaluate what you have learned from this unit and to demonstrate to what extent you now understand the basic terminology of research and the principles of research design.

Session objectives

When you have completed this session you should be able to:

- carry out a critical review of a research article

- define the basic terminology used in research activity

- identify why a knowledge of research is useful to you in your own field of study.

1: Critical reading of research findings

When we talk about 'critical reading' what we mean is using the knowledge you have gained in working through this text to question and challenge what you read in research reports. We hope by this stage you will be able to use your knowledge to judge why particular approaches to research were adopted by the researcher.

In Session Two we gave you a broad framework that indicated the 'research process', as follows:

1   Identify a research problem.

2   Read the literature pertaining to the problem.

3   Design the study.

4   Collect the data.

5   Analyse the data and present the findings.

6   Compare the findings with the original literature.

7   Draw conclusions and make recommendations.

8   Present a written report.

To consider whether the findings from a research project can be generalised to a variety of situations, you need to use the knowledge you have gained of the research process to challenge the findings of the research.

ACTIVITY 54   ALLOW 60 MINUTES

Choose and reread one of the research articles that you selected for your literature review in Session Two. Now that you have had an opportunity to explore in more depth the issues we introduced to you then, we want you to undertake a more critical appraisal than you did earlier.

On a separate sheet write down your answers to the following questions in relation to each stage of the research reported in the article you have selected. It may help you to use the framework we outlined in *Table 2.2* in Session Two.

Start by asking yourself at the outset whether the report was presented in a clear, logical and unambiguous way. Then go on to address the following issues.

1   *Research problem*

   ● are the research aims and the hypothesis or question clearly stated?

2   *The literature pertaining to the problem*

   ● is there clear evidence that the author has read the literature relevant to the field of study?

   ● is this literature review up to date?

   ● has the author used the findings from the literature to design his or her research?

3 *Ethical issues*

   ● were any ethical issues anticipated – if yes, how were these resolved?

4 *Research design*

   ● what is the overall study design (quantitative or qualitative)?

   ● what sampling procedures were used?

   ● how were the research tools developed?

   ● was reliability/validity considered?

   ● is there any evidence of bias in the design?

5 *Data collection*

   ● how were the data collected ?

   ● what steps were taken to ensure the reliability and validity of the data collected?

   ● is there any evidence of bias at this stage?

6 *Analysis of the data and presentation of the findings*

   ● how were the data analysed?

   ● is there any evidence of bias or misrepresentation in the data analysis?

   ● are the findings presented clearly and logically?

7 *The findings*

   ● are the findings linked with the literature review in such a way as to support or refute the findings from other studies?

8 *Conclusions and recommendations*

   ● how did the author draw conclusions from the research?

   ● are any limitations or underlying assumptions in the research design noted?

In view of the overall findings from the research do you feel that the findings have any relevance to your own area of practice?

Commentary

We expect you were able to approach this exercise more critically than you did in Session Two as you have now had an opportunity to explore the range of issues in more detail. We also anticipate that the article you read was not 'perfect' on every count. Once you have a clear idea of the steps in the research process it is much easier to identify areas where researchers have not clearly spelled out aspects of their research.

1 Even at the beginning of an article it is not always clear exactly what a researcher intends to do and the aims of their research may not be obvious.

2 When looking at the literature review there might be evidence to indicate that the researcher has read a lot of other research related to a project. However, in published research reports this is often presented in a very abbreviated form – you may have felt that you wanted to know more about what the literature showed in your article.

3 It is not always clearly indicated how researchers approach the ethical dilemmas their research generates – they may take them for granted, but this does not help the reader who may have a particular wish to know about them.

4&5 When looking at the different stages of the research process you might have found that the authors gave a very clear account of some aspects but a not so clear account of others. The researcher might have noted clearly how the data were collected but spent little time discussing analysis. Conversely, they may have spent a lot of time discussing the analysis of the data but not clearly illustrated how they collected the data.

6&7 It is important to ensure that the findings from the research are accurately recorded. If they are not clearly spelled out, or perhaps are inadequately presented, the reader may be none the wiser at the end of the report than at the beginning. Clarity of presentation is critical in research results.

8 Finally, it is important that you are sure that the conclusions and recommendations are based on the research findings presented. It is possible for bias to be introduced, even at this late stage of the research report, if researchers do not take care to focus on what they *have* found rather than on what they thought they *should have* found.

As any research report forms part of a wider context, in our case health and social care, it is important that findings are linked to existing knowledge – perhaps supporting findings from other studies or refuting them. It is the *collective* picture of research findings that will help us to determine whether we should be reviewing our practices in the light of the research findings. This is a very practical point, as it demonstrates how difficult it is to change your practice on the basis of only one or two written reports. Unless you are absolutely convinced about the reliability and validity of a research study, you would be very unwise to change practice on the basis of one small report.

It would now be useful for you to try this exercise again with several different articles. This will give you a good idea how different components of research are explained by different researchers in published research. However, when you are doing this take care that you are judging the contents of the article – not the researcher! Whenever a research report is written, the researcher has to make decisions about what to include in the sometimes limited space available for publication. As we noted above, if you find there is not enough information about a subject, you will need to search out more literature to build up your knowledge base.

2: The basic terminology used in research activity

The next section involves a self-test activity. A list of research terms has been provided and you are asked to write down what you consider to be an appropriate definition or explanation for each term. You are advised to do this from memory initially, but if you find difficulty with any term it is recommended that you review Sessions One to Five until you find the relevant term. You can check your definitions and explanations by referring to the Glossary of Key Concepts at the end of the text.

ACTIVITY 55   ALLOW 45 MINUTES

Define the following terms in your own words.

Term	
CD-Rom	
Convenience sample	
Data collection techniques	
Dependent variable	
Descriptive design	
Descriptive statistics	
Evaluation research	
Hypothesis	

Independent variable	
Inferential statistics	
Literature review	
Mean	
Median	
Mode	
Observation	
Population	
Purposive sample	
Qualitative research methods	
Quantitative research methods	
Random sample	
Range	

Reliability	
Research design	
Sample	
Validity	
Variable	

Commentary

If you were able to complete the list of definitions above from memory you obviously have a good grasp of the core knowledge required to begin a more in-depth study of specific aspects of research.

If you had difficulties, go back and re-read the relevant part of the text and then retest yourself on another day.

We would now like you to consider further the implications of studying research in the context of your own professional role or area of work. We suggest that your final activity should be a review of the reasons why you feel, on conclusion of this unit, that research is important in your area of study.

ACTIVITY 56 ALLOW 25 MINUTES

Write at least 100 words summarising why a knowledge of research is important to you in your area of practice.

Commentary

Professional practitioners today can no longer allow care to be carried out in an unquestioning manner. We live and work in a world that challenges the basis of our professional practice and asks us to demonstrate the outcomes of the care we offer. If we are to prove to colleagues and managers that our care is effective, we need some understanding of how to go about it. We need to be able to critically read research related to our own areas. It is only by doing so that we can develop effective practice informed by recent research.

Summary

In Session Six you have explored:

1 The meaning of 'critical reading'.

2 How to use the knowledge gained about the research process to challenge the context of research articles.

3 Basic research terminology.

Check that you have achieved the objectives given at the beginning of this session and, if not, review the appropriate sections. You may now wish to progress to one of our other units in this series to explore some of the issues mentioned in this core unit in more detail.

LEARNING REVIEW

You can use the list of learning outcomes given below to review the progress you have made during this unit: the list is a repeat of the one provided at the beginning. You should tick the box on the scale that corresponds most closely to the point you feel you have achieved now and then compare it with your scores on the learning profile completed at the beginning of the unit. If there are any areas that you are still unsure about, you might like to review the session concerned.

	Not at all	Partly	Quite well	Very well

Session One

I can:

- explain the nature and benefits of research-based practice in health and social care   ☐ ☐ ☐ ☐
- identify specific areas of my practice which need to be researched   ☐ ☐ ☐ ☐
- explain the basic questions which should inform any research.   ☐ ☐ ☐ ☐

Session Two

I can:

- define the meaning of terms commonly used in research   ☐ ☐ ☐ ☐
- use an academic or professional library   ☐ ☐ ☐ ☐
- carry out a basic literature review.   ☐ ☐ ☐ ☐

Session Three

I can:

- distinguish between the differing approaches adopted in quantitative and qualitative research   ☐ ☐ ☐ ☐
- outline different ways in which data can be collected   ☐ ☐ ☐ ☐
- explain the meaning of the 'population' and the 'sample'.   ☐ ☐ ☐ ☐

Session Four

I can:

- explain the concepts of reliability and validity in research   ☐ ☐ ☐ ☐

	Not at all	Partly	Quite well	Very well

Session Four *continued*

- describe what is meant by 'indirect' and 'direct' sources of data $\square$ $\square$ $\square$ $\square$
- state the differences between the data collected in a quantitative study and the data collected in a qualitative study. $\square$ $\square$ $\square$ $\square$

Session Five

I can:

- state what is meant by the terms mean, range, median, mode, standard deviation $\square$ $\square$ $\square$ $\square$
- describe the first step in qualitative data analysis $\square$ $\square$ $\square$ $\square$
- explain the purpose of using statistics in data analysis. $\square$ $\square$ $\square$ $\square$

Session Six

I can:

- carry out a critical review of a research article $\square$ $\square$ $\square$ $\square$
- define the basic terminology used in research activity $\square$ $\square$ $\square$ $\square$
- identify why a knowledge of research is useful in my own field of study. $\square$ $\square$ $\square$ $\square$

RESOURCES SECTION

Contents

RESOURCE I

Howard, R. (1995)
Nursing Times,
March 29,
Vol.91, No.13,
pp. 40–43.

Reasons for older people attending A&E

Editor's comment

We live in a society in which the population is gradually ageing. We are reminded by Rita Howard's article that the majority of older people are living in the community, thus raising the issue of how responsive health and social services are to older people's needs at times of perceived crisis or health breakdown. A lack of accessible services may lead to older people using A & E departments.

It might be that as a consequence we witness the emergence of older people viewed as a group of unpopular patients, being seen as making unjustifiable visits to A & E departments. The challenge must be to explore the specialist needs of these people to ensure that they are no longer marginalised. Health and social care staff need expertise in their area of work with a sound application of this knowledge to the care of this population.

Gordon Evans, MSc, RMN, RGN, RNT, FETC, is senior tutor in post-basic care, North Yorkshire College of Health.

Key words: older people, A. & E, discharge planning

Abstract

This study aimed to identify any shortfalls in the discharge of older people from an A & E department and areas in which improvements could be made.

The findings highlighted the fact that more than 40% of the attendances to A & E did not require urgent treatment and that nearly 59% of attenders lived alone.

The terms 'justifiable' and 'unjustifiable', applied to attendances in the study group, are used in this paper to differentiate between cases where immediate attention was required and where it was not. This judgement was based on the author's professional knowledge (see discussion section).

It is frequently suggested by health professionals that a large proportion of the population aged 75 years and over are increasingly attending A & E departments inappropriately. We therefore conducted a three-month study to follow up patients in this age group discharged from Whipps Cross A & E department, London.

The aim of our study was to assess whether the A & E department was able to help them, whether patients' problems had

been dealt with adequately and whether they were coping at home following discharge. The need for further action was also explored.

Our assessment was based primarily on the patient's perspective of how he or she was coping after discharge. In some cases, we contacted the main carer involved, that is, the district nurse, the home-care attendant or the patient's relative.

Method

Basic data regarding the patient's medical history and his or her reason for attendance were obtained from the casualty card.

We noted date and time of attendance, the presenting diagnosis and action taken in respect of referrals and treatment. Some patients had been in-patients before, and we consulted our own record cards for further information.

Following this data collection we subsequently contacted each patient or carer, usually by telephone, to inquire about his or her progress. Where there was no telephone we visited the patient at home. All information was recorded in a ledger for further reference.

Results

The total number of people involved in the study was 364, of whom 118 (32.4%) were men and 246 (67.5%) women. Of these, 213 (67.5%) people lived alone (51 men and 161 women). Contact was not established with 18 (4.94%). Eight had reattended and been admitted to hospital and the remaining 10 failed to respond to telephone calls and home visits. Further intervention was necessary in three cases. The first was a woman with a post-operative eye problem living alone who seemed very negative about her circumstances and was referred to a social worker. The second was a woman whose mobility had deteriorated rapidly over two weeks; she was referred to the hospital occupational therapist, who arranged to visit her at home. A third woman lived alone and had arthritis. She had the added complication of arm and leg injuries which limited her activities of daily living, so a referral was made for occupational therapy assessment.

In all, 60.7% (221) of visits were 'justifiable' in our estimation, based on the limited information at our disposal. Living alone did not significantly affect the ratio between 'justified' and 'unjustified' attendances (*Fig 1*).

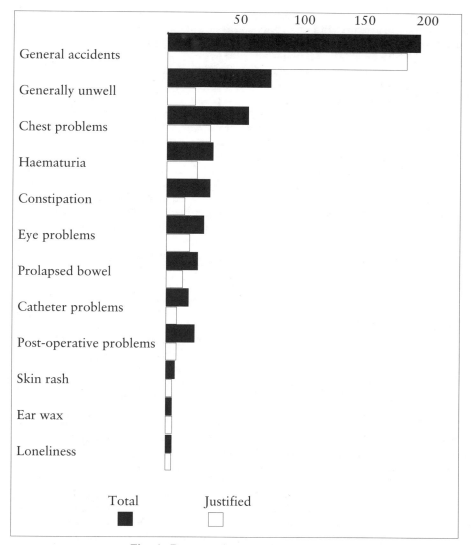

Fig. 1: Reasons for attendance

The majority (80%) of justifiable attendances were in the general accident category, as would be expected. Of the four visits that were not justifiable, one was a simple faint, two were habitual attenders (one had an old fracture of the nose and the other was living alone and was unhappy about it); the fourth had injured her leg a week before the visit.

Chest problems accounted for 18 justifiable attendances, and these were mostly chest pains. The vast number of unjustifiable visits in this category were chronic conditions and, of the remainder, three had been recently bereaved, one had experienced a panic attack, one stated the GP was not supportive and another said his GP was on holiday.

Seven justifiable visits were in the haemorrhage group and these were prolonged epistaxis (one woman attended three times before being seen by an ENT specialist). The unjustifiable attendances were three people with self-resolving epistaxis, four with haematuria, one with a problematic colostomy, one with rectal bleeding, one who had vomited after a meal owing to gastritis and one who had a long-standing lump on the cheek.

Of the eight generally unwell patients who constituted justifiable visits, two were GP referrals for possible admission, one (with a possible carcinoma) who refused admission and the other was immobile and sent home without an occupational therapy assessment. Two in this category had pain, one related to a soft tissue injury and the other was concerned about his pacemaker. One woman had gone missing for several hours from respite care and the remaining three were a patient with known angina complaining of pins and needles, a patient with a possible deep vein thrombosis and a patient with an atrial fibrillation for ECG. The unjustifiable attenders in this category mainly had general aches and pains that should have been seen by a GP and, if necessary, been referred to an out-patients department. One man admitted that he was simply seeking a second opinion on his knee pain.

There were six post-operative problems,

four of which were justifiable visits in that one required resuturing and two had haematomas. The two unjustifiable visits were post-operative swelling in one patient, but it is perhaps understandable that a patient would return to hospital rather than consult a GP following an operation.

Nine patients attended with eye problems, four of which we could justify in that one was a post-operative problem, one had a foreign body in the eye, one had sudden loss of vision and the other had put cat ear drops into her eyes and was referred by her GP for an emergency check. The unjustifiable visits consisted of blurred vision, black spots, pressure, possible infection and a non-specific problem.

Of the six catheter/urinary problems we found three justifiable visits. The justifiable attendances involved two indwelling catheters that fell out, one at night, while another had carcinoma of the prostate and bones; the other patient had retention of urine. The unjustifiable visits involved two indwelling catheters; one patient had an infection and required antibiotics, the other catheter fell out and the patient did not contact the district nurse. The last patient in this group was complaining of dysuria and did not have a catheter.

Of the three visits involving rashes, one was justifiable in that it involved cellulitis with secondary conjunctivitis and occurred on a Sunday. The two unjustifiable visits involved one allergic rash; the other needed only to be referred to the dermatologist by the GP, but the patient's son said he was unhappy with their doctor.

We decided that the 12 constipation cases were all unjustifiable, as all were relieved by enemata, bulk-forming laxatives and other interventions that could have been performed by GPs. This was also true of the bowel prolapses, eight in all, as these were reducible and/or required referral via the out-patients' department. The one ear problem, registered as a foreign body in the ear, was found to involve excessive ear wax. We therefore concluded that the GP could have arranged for syringeing without recourse to the A & E department.

As for the man who came in because he was lonely, he frequently visited the department and died at home in January.

Discussion

Whipps Cross Hospital has one of the busiest A & E departments in London[1]. None the less it maintains a good discharge record of patients aged 75 and over[11]. The department of medicine for older people accepts all patients aged 75 and over with medical problems and other problems such as upper limb fractures. The hospital also has an observation ward where patients can be admitted overnight and assessed for discharge or transfer to another ward. The A & E department has an occupational therapist based on site to carry out immediate assessments, a resource not always available in most other hospitals; this person plays a large part in the decision to admit or discharge.

It became fairly obvious to us that problems were not so much about how the patient is dealt with in the A & E department, but more about the reason they attend in the first place. Because this seemed a substantial issue, given our remit to highlight any problems, we decided to look more closely at so-called 'unjustified' attendances to the department. We realise this is a controversial area and one that depends on hindsight and involves an element of subjectivity.

Conclusion

Even if a large proportion of the population aged 75 and over attends A & E departments inappropriately it is necessary to keep a sense of proportion; as Montalvo et al.[6] point out: 'This group of patients tends to use the service more adequately than younger adults (since they go to A & E with more justifiable reason, with more severe diseases and require more hospital admissions), but they do consume proportionately more time.' As Buechner observes: 'The largest age group attending A & E are 25–44 years';[7] thus the age group covered by this study must be seen as a minor part of a larger issue (Box 1).

As a large percentage live alone, this suggests that social isolation may play a big part in this problem, as a number of researchers have concluded.[3-6] It is necessary to consider that the dying process must also have implications in many of the presenting problems and perhaps the underlying message may be an anxiety about dying in isolation. Certainly many people expressed pleasure at receiving a follow-up check. We feel there is a place for continued follow-up of this particularly vulnerable group in the light of these observations. Several people were given advice regarding social support and guidance on appropriate action to take if problems arose.

Health visitors who work with older people are looking at ways to develop their service and have shown an interest in our study. They certainly seem to be ideally suited to visit patients following A & E attendance to pick up on underlying issues and problems and to refer to appropriate agencies. Often a home visit may bring to light something a patient is reluctant to talk about in a more formal setting. We have all experienced cases of older people who struggle on in difficult circumstances not knowing (and sometimes not wanting to know) how to get support. Failing this, there may be an opportunity for hospital liaison sisters to develop their role in this direction. We are therefore hopeful that a follow-up scheme will be devised in the future.

Limitations of the study

It was obvious during our study that no checklist was being used. In the light of such a good discharge record it is possible that in a fast-moving A & E department such a checklist is considered a burden. It would, however, be useful for further reference should a problem arise after discharge.

Implications for practice

This study, like others,[2-6] has clarified the fact that the underlying problem with all attenders, especially the population aged 75 and over, is not so much about how they are discharged from A & E departments but, rather, how they use such departments. Various solutions have been proposed, including increased health education for older people,[2,4] more information and better facilities for GPs,[2,4] improved integration between A & E departments, GPs and social services [2,3] and appropriate staff training in dealing with older people.[3] One study [5] suggests staffing levels should be adjusted according to fluctuations in the demand on A & E and another [6] that appropriate facilities be provided for older people.

Health education is widely recognised as essential, not least with the older population. This could be approached by running sessions at day-care facilities and drop-in centres. Videotapes could be shown and perhaps television programmes aimed at older people. A good investment for the future would be for more preventive work in schools and colleges to be initiated.

It is evident that there are still problems at GP level to be addressed. Perhaps some education among this group about appro-

priate referral systems would be valuable.

We feel that a good way of integrating community care with the A & E department is to bring these under the same roof by having a GP surgery on site. Perhaps having a social worker on site and therefore available for consultation would enhance this integration process further. On the other hand, some researchers, on finding that much abuse stems from non-willingness to use the GP service for a variety of reasons, felt that providing GP cover in an A & E department would only open the floodgates to more abuse.[9] They suggest that triage nurses should be the key figures in the re-education of the public in appropriate A & E use.

Green and Dale[9] also talk about GP dissatisfaction and lack of facilities and observe that social deprivation and distance from hospital play a part in 'inappropriate' attendances. They open up the discussion to include staff attitudes leading to labelling of patients as inappropriate attenders. Their study highlighted moral evaluations made on the basis of superficial appearances as well as presenting medical problems. They also make a very valid point that 'a major shortcoming in much of the research has been that 'inappropriate' patients have generally been labelled through retrospective comparison with 'legitimate' patients'.

It is easy for us to make judgements after the fact, as pointed out by Green and Dale. For the patient 'a rational response to unfamiliar symptoms is to be cautious and consider the worst possible scenario until this is excluded'. Like us they conclude that 'the most productive policy may be to provide appropriate care rather than attempt to deflect such care to the community'.

We have a population that is ageing. Although this group constitutes a relatively

---

Box 1. Recommendations and implications for practice

- There is a need for more education regarding use of the A & E department and what other referral systems are appropriate to the condition of the patient.

- District nurses must ensure that all patients with indwelling catheters are aware that when a problem arises the first line of contact should be the district nurse.

- A GP surgery on site in the A & E department and run by local GPs on a rota basis could help to relieve the burden of inappropriate attendances.

- There seems to be a place for health visitors to follow up this population of particularly vulnerable people and perhaps hospital liaison sisters could help with this.

- Patients being discharged from surgical wards could benefit by receiving written information regarding what to do should complications arise.

small population of attenders at A & E departments, they require more intensive health care attention than they obtain at present.

Key points

- A large percentage of older people attending A & E departments may have conditions which could be easily treated by their general practitioners
- Many of the older people whose attendances might be classified as 'inappropriate' live alone
- Health visitors could play an important part in ensuring that older people receive appropriate treatment, reducing the load on already stretched A & E departments
- Checklists could be useful in ensuring that older people are discharged from A & E departments with an assurance of adequate follow-up
- Further research into 'unjustifiable' attendances is essential

References

1   Davison, A. G., Hildren, A.C.C., Floyer, M.A,. Use and misuse of an accident and emergency department in the East End of London *Journal of the Royal Society of Medicine*, 1983; **76**: 37–40.
2   Dove, A .F., Dave, S. H. Elderly patients in the accident and emergency department and their problems. *British Medical Journal*, 1986; **292**: 807–809.
3   Davies, T. Accident department or general practice? *British Medical Journal*, 1986; **292**: 6515, 242–243.
4   Williams, E., Pottle, B. The ups and downs of accident and emergency. *Nursing Times* 1989, **85**: 47, 60–64
5   Wood, J. Elderly people in accident and emergency. *Nursing Times,* 1992; **88**: 3, 63–65.
6   Gonzalez Montalvo, J .I., Elosua de Juan, I., Guillen Llera, F. The elderly patient in the emergency service: some myths and some answers. *Rivesta Clinica Espanola* 1990; **87**: 7, 348–352.
7   Buechner, J. S. Use of hospital emergency departments for routine medical care. *Rhode Island Medical Journal* 1991; **74**: 9, 434–435.
8   Foroughin, D., Chadwick, L. Accident and emergency abusers. *Practitioner* 1989; **233**: 1468, 657–659.
9   Green, J., Dale, J. Primary care in accident and emergency and general practice: a comparison. *Social Science and Medicine* 1992; **35**: 987–995.
10 Howard, R., Heeks, A., Friel, M. Return to hospital, *Journal of District Nursing* 1991; **10**: 2, 8–10.

RESOURCE 2

Firn, S. (1995)
Nursing Times,
February 22,
Vol.91, No.8,
pp. 37–39

Psychological and emotional impact of an HIV diagnosis

Stephen Firn, BSc, MSc, RMN, is a lecturer/practitioner in HIV and mental health at the Bethlem and Maudsley NHS Trust and is seconded half-time to the RCN as community health advisor with specialist lead in HIV, community health and infection control. Ian F Norman, BA, MSc, PhD, RMN, is a senior lecturer and director of post-graduate studies, Department of Nursing Studies, King's College, University of London.

Key words: HIV/AIDS, user views, psychological needs, emotional needs, impact of illness

Abstract

This is the first of two papers that reports the results of a research study into the psychological and emotional needs of people with HIV and how nurses might best offer support. This paper discusses the psychological impact of HIV diagnosis. Inductive analysis of in-depth interviews with in-patients and their nurses generated five themes: reactions to critical events related to HIV infection; changes in body image and chronic ill health; fear and rejection; cognitive and minor dysfunctions associated with HIV; and absent friends.

HIV has been associated with the development of a range of mental health problems. Although some of these are common to other life threatening illnesses, people with HIV infection and AIDS may experience psychosocial and neuropsychiatric disturbances which are specifically related to their knowledge of being infected, as well as to the direct effects of the virus.

Identified psychiatric disorders in HIV

include acute stress reactions; adjustment disorders; functional psychoses such as depression and schizophreniform disorders; and suicidal ideas and attempts.

Many of these disorders have been linked to the stresses and losses associated with living with the virus. Triggers include the uncertainty surrounding disease progression and outcomes, the distressing nature of the symptoms themselves and the knowledge that HIV is a potentially fatal disease. In addition, many of those affected are relatively young people who are often least prepared for such illnesses; their lifestyles may have been stigmatised before the advent of HIV (for example gay men, drug users, prostitutes); and people who have experienced chronic ill health (such as people with haemophilia).[5-7]

The ways in which AIDS has become the focus for societal prejudices and concerns have been well documented.[8,9] It follows that after a positive HIV antibody test, many people must not only come to terms with the implications of the diagnosis, but must also cope with the potentially negative reactions of partners, friends, family and other social contacts. This may mean that people with HIV disease feel unable to seek social support, or find that support is not forthcoming and this is likely to exacerbate any existing mental health problems.

HIV has also been shown to cause a variety of acute and chronic neuropsychiatric (organic) disorders which arise from two types of pathological processes. The virus can directly affect the brain and central nervous system (CNS) causing a dementia-type illness characterised by progressive cognitive and/or motor impairment which may be accompanied by behavioural disturbances.[11,12] Alternatively, neuropsychiatric functioning may be impaired by opportunistic infections and/or neoplasms affecting the CNS.

It is not clear how widespread mental health problems are among people with HIV. Although researchers have attempted to collect epidemiological data on this topic, wide variations have emerged due to methodological limitations of the research studies. These include heavy reliance on anecdotal case reports, lack of comparability between the measures used and an absence of a suitable control group.

Further, many studies have been conducted by psychiatrists or neurologists who base their findings on people with HIV who are referred to them. These studies have reported high levels of psychosocial and neuropsychiatric disorders, but it is unwise to extrapolate from these findings.[3] But the continued spread of HIV and improved treatment and prophylaxis, which ensures that people with HIV live longer, mean the incidence of HIV-related neurological dysfunctions is likely to increase. Here we present

our research: see Box 1 for methods and Box 2 overleaf for findings.

Box 1 Methods

In an attempt to increase our understanding of these issues we conducted an exploratory study, which sought to describe how patients with AIDS, and their nurses, perceived the emotional and psychological issues faced by people with AIDS, and the nurses' role in responding to these issues.

Focused interviews were conducted with an opportunistic sample of patients and nurses of one general hospital ward in which 50% of the beds were reserved for people with AIDS-related illness. A total of seven patients (five men and two women), all of whom had a clinical diagnosis of AIDS, and 10 registered general nurses (two men and eight women) were interviewed. The nurses represented different grades (D–F) and had worked in the ward between five weeks and seven years. The patients included gay and straight men and drug users who had been inpatients for between eight days and eight weeks. Six patients had previously been admitted to the ward.

The interviews, which lasted between 45 and 90 minutes, were audio-tape recorded with the respondents' permission and transcribed for analysis. Analysis involved inductive categorisation of the interview data to generate themes which comprehensively summarised the data.

Since data collection was restricted to one site and more information could have been obtained from further interviews, the results cannot be considered generalisable. Nevertheless, they provide a valuable insight into the perceptions of nurses and people with AIDS in this ward at the time of the study.

The interviews focused on two questions which were subjected to a slight amendment when the respondent was a nurse rather than a patient. The patients' questions were:

- What have you found to be the main emotional and psychological issues you have had to face since discovering you were infected with HIV?
- What do you consider to be the nurse's role in responding to the emotional and psychological issues that you have described?

This article discusses responses to the first of these questions only.

Box 2 Findings

An analysis of the respondents' perceptions of the emotional and psychological issues faced by people with HIV yielded five themes:

- Reactions to critical events related to HIV infection

- Changes in body images and chronic ill health
- Fear and rejection: the social construction of AIDS
- Cognitive and minor dysfunctions associated with HIV
- Absent friends: the death of loved ones through AIDS.

Reactions to critical events related to infection

A number of critical events describing when people with HIV may be most at risk of experiencing emotional and psychological distress were listed. For example, all the respondents identified the time immediately following the HIV diagnosis as being particularly traumatic. This is not surprising and is a common finding in relation to other potentially serious illnesses. However, patients also described other periods of potential crisis which may be less well recognised. One of these was the initial admission to hospital: the respondent described her feelings of horror when she was admitted to the ward and saw other people with AIDS for the first time. She said: 'God was I in a state. Not when I first heard about being positive because I knew there was something wrong. But I didn't realise what a terrible illness it is. I mean, the other patients looked like something out of Belsen'.

This woman's distress was heightened because she was admitted at night and nobody explained to her why she was in hospital and what was going to happen. Such was her distress that she took an overdose when she returned home. Thus, in some cases, it seems that admission to hospital and being confronted with the realities of AIDS may be more traumatic than receiving the initial HIV diagnosis.

The moment when a person receives an AIDS diagnosis was also seen as crucial since a number of patients said that they had learned to cope with being HIV positive by convincing themselves that they were not going to develop AIDS. One patient said he used to think: 'I won't get AIDS. Everyone else gets AIDS. I know I'm HIV positive but I haven't had any illnesses so why should I go on to get AIDS?'

This patient was completely unprepared for being told of his diagnosis and felt that the nurse informed him in a rather casual manner that his physical condition had deteriorated to the extent that he now had AIDS. The nurse seems to have incorrectly assumed that he was prepared for this news and would be able to cope.

What these critical events indicate, is that just because a person has known of his or her HIV status for some time, he or she will not necessarily be prepared for what will happen if he or she becomes unwell. This indicates

the value of mental health nurses being available to offer time and support to help patients adjust to further loss and change.

Changes in body image and chronic ill health

Changes in body image was identified by patients as a source of much emotional distress. One respondent graphically described his feelings as follows: 'It is about accepting how your life changes. Throwing up every night or every morning. Or having bad diarrhoea. Or not eating anything and just losing lots of weight. Yes, I get freaked out. There was a stage when my hair was coming out. I thought "I don't want to be bald at 30. This is a bit much".'

An instrument designed to identify people who are at risk of developing a seriously altered body image[17] identifies three important components: body reality; body presentation; and body ideal.

Body reality refers to the areas of the body which are altered in appearance with changes in the face, hands and sexual organs having potential for causing the greatest distress. These seem to be the areas most affected in HIV disease. For instance, a number of respondents spoke of the effects of Kaposi's sarcoma, a type of skin cancer that commonly affects the face, and which one respondent said made her feel like 'a leper'. Other respondents described the very visible effects of weight loss and the distressing effects of repeated infections in the genital areas, such as herpes and thrush.

Body presentation relates to ways in which the body functions. Patients interviewed repeatedly mentioned incontinence as being a particularly distressing loss of bodily control. A number also spoke of the frustration of being unable to complete tasks requiring physical exertion or mental concentration, which they had found easy in the past.

Body ideal relates to people's perceptions of how they expect their body to appear and function. As some people with AIDS are relatively young, it is reasonable to assume that generally they have high expectations from life and so are somewhat less prepared for debilitating illness than people with other potentially life threatening conditions.

These findings suggest that people with AIDS may be at high risk of experiencing psychological distress as a result of changes in their body image. The extent of this distress was underestimated by nurses interviewed in the study and this is reflected in the AIDS literature. Although Price's instrument[17] was not developed specifically for people with HIV, it seems to offer a promising assessment measure.

Fear and rejection: social construction of AIDS

Respondents described how the sympathy and support that someone with a life-threatening illness might reasonably expect from friends and relatives, was sometimes withheld in their case. One patient had been forced to leave his job as a care worker for people with learning disabilities because his colleagues refused to work with him.

AIDS is potentially stigmatising because people with it are often perceived as having engaged in activities which may be proscribed by society and, by implication, of belonging to a stigmatised group such as gay men or drug users. These beliefs are often exhibited in the language of blame – social attitudes to which nurses are not immune as illustrated in the following extract from a nurse's interview: 'As I said about blood transfusions, I don't know if innocent is the right word, but they are kind of victims, you know? It's not their fault they became infected.'

This shows that even nurses who have chosen to work in specialist wards caring for people with AIDS can have difficulties in viewing their patients completely non-judgementally.

Cognitive and minor dysfunctions

Fears about developing cognitive impairment were expressed by a number of patients. Some even said they felt they had come to terms with the prospect of their impending death, but could not contemplate 'losing their minds'.

One patient looked around the ward and said: 'I think when people (with AIDS) are mentally ill they should be put to sleep. When they are totally ga ga and don't know what's going on. I mean, what is their quality of life?'

Clearly there is a role here for nurses to provide patients with accurate information about HIV-associated dementia, to help them explore their fears, assist them to make decisions about their care and attend to unfinished business which they may be unable to see to in the future. Mental health nurses are well-placed to carry out these functions.

There is also a need for interventions developed in relation to older people with dementia to be adapted to promote the quality of life of people with AIDS who have a cognitive impairment.

Absent friends: the death of loved ones

The final theme, the loss of loved ones from AIDS, was identified by a number of patients as an additional stress which heightened fears about their own mortality. One respondent spoke very movingly of seeing his friends and associates die one by one. He felt unable to cope with attending another funeral.

Some important insights were gained from this study regarding nurses' and AIDS patients' perceptions of the emotional and psychological issues facing people with HIV. All respondents were aware of the potentially traumatic effects of receiving a HIV positive diagnosis, and this is recognised in the literature.[18]

However, patients' descriptions of their experiences drew attention to other crisis periods such as when physical symptoms first occur or worsen; admission to an AIDS ward; and when people first receive an AIDS diagnosis. People's abilities to adapt to change and loss seemed to be related to their previous coping mechanisms and perceived levels of social support, although patients did not support the view of some nurses that perceived high-risk behaviour prior to infection is an important determinant of the need for emotional and psychological support.

All the respondents were concerned about the distressing changes in body image that people with AIDS experience. Many are young with strong ambitions and a high social status prior to the illness. The impact of these changes seems to be underestimated in the HIV literature and further research is required to explore the extent to which change in body image is a significant factor in the emotional and psychological distress of this patient group.

The effects of the social stigma that surrounds HIV have been extensively documented[19] and were reported by almost all respondents. Moral panic theory has been widely used to explain the mass of societal responses to the syndrome.[20] However, it cannot explain why some patients, who acquired the virus through heterosexual intercourse or infected blood transfusions, did not identify with gay men with AIDS, and even blamed them for causing their infection.

Goffman provides a plausible explanation in his analysis of stigma: 'Such an individual has thoroughly learned about the normal and the stigmatised long before he must see himself as deficient. Presumably he will have a special problem in reinventing himself, and a special likelihood of developing disapproval of self.' [21]

This insight is important since as HIV infection continues to increase through heterosexual intercourse, services will need to diversify and recognise that people with HIV do not form a homogenous group with identical needs.

References

1   Maj, M. Psychiatric aspects of HIV – infection and AIDS. *Psychological Medicine* 1990; **20**: 3, 547–563.

2   Catalan, J. Psychosocial and neuropsy-

chiatric aspects of HIV infection: review of their extent and implications for psychiatry. *Psychosomatic Research* 1988; **32**: 3, 237–248.

3 Atkinson, J., Grant, I., Kennedy, C.J. et al. Prevalence of psychiatric disorders among men infected with human immunodeficiency virus. *Archives of General Psychiatry* 1988; **45**: 8, 859–864.

4 Marzuk, P.M., Tierney, H., Tardiff, K. et al. Increased risk of suicide in persons with AIDS. *Journal of the American Medical Association* 1988; **259**: 9,1333.

5 Catalan, J., Riccio, M. Brain damage and psychiatric hospital closures: a policy rethink. *Psychiatric Bulletin* 1990; **14**: 694–696.

6 Miller, D., Riccio, M. Non-organic psychiatric and psychosocial syndromes associated with HIV-1 infection and disease. *AIDS* 1990; **4**: 381–388.

7 King, M.B. Psychological aspects of HIV infection and AIDS: what have we learned? *British Journal of Psychiatry* 1990; **156**: 2, 151–156.

8 Weeks, J. Love in a cold climate. In Aggleton, P., Homans, H. (eds). *Social Aspects of AIDS*. Lewes: The Falmer Press, 1988.

9 Patton, C. *Sex and Germs: the Politics of AIDS*. Boston: South End Press, 1985.

10 Aggleton, P., Homans, H., Mojsa, J. et al. *AIDS: Scientific and Social Issues*. Edinburgh: Churchill Livingstone, 1989.

11 Maj, M. Organic mental disorders in HIV infection. *AIDS* 1990; **4**: 831–840.

12 Everall, I.P., Luthert, P.J., Lantos, P.L. Neuronal loss in the frontal cortex in HIV infection. *Lancet* 1991; **337**: 8750, 1119–1121.

13 McAllister, R.H., Harrison, M.J.G. HIV and the nervous system. *Brit. Journ. Hosp. Med.* 1988: July: 21–26.

14 Vogel-Sciblia, S.E., Mulsant, B.H., Keshavan, M.S. HIV infection presenting as psychosis: a critique. *Acta Psychiatry Scandinavia* 1988; **78**: 652–656.

15 Halstead, S., Riccio, M., Harlow, P., Oretti, R., Thompson, C. Psychosis associated with HIV infection. *British Journal of Psychiatry* 1988; **153**: 5, 618–623.

16 Kocsis, A. Review of neuropsychological studies of HIV infection. *AIDS Care* 1990; **2**: 4, 385–388.

17 Price, B. *Body Image: Nursing Concepts and Care*. Hemel Hempstead: Prentice Hall, 1990.

18 Miller, D., Bor, R. *AIDS: A Guide to Clinical Counselling*. London: Science Press, 1988.

19 Aggleton, P., Homans, H., Mojsa, J. et al. *AIDS: Scientific and Social Issues*. Edinburgh: Churchill Livingstone, 1988.

20 Small, N. Aids and Social Policy. *Critical Social Policy*. 1988; Spring: 9–29.

21 Goffman, E. *Stigma*. Harmondsworth: Penguin, 1990.

This is the second article of a series on HIV. The first article was published on January 11 and the next will appear on March 22.

FURTHER READING

AUDIT COMMISSION (1993) *Children First: A study of hospital services*, HMSO, London.

BOWLBY, J (1951) *Maternal Care and Mental Health*, WHO, Geneva.

CLARKE, E (1991) *Research Awareness: A programme for nurses, midwives and health visitors*, Distance Learning Centre, South Bank Polytechnic.

CLIFFORD, C and GOUGH, S (1990) *Nursing Research: A skills-based introduction*, Prentice Hall.

DEALY, C (1994) *The Care of Wounds – A Guide for Nursing*, Blackwell Scientific.

DEPARTMENT OF HEALTH (1991) *The Health of the Nation*, HMSO, London.

DEPARTMENT OF HEALTH (1989) *Caring for People: Community care in the next decade and beyond*, Cm. 849, HMSO.

DEPARTMENT OF HEALTH (1983) *NHS Management Inquiry*, (Chair: R. Griffiths) HMSO, London.

FIRN, S and NORMAN, I (1995) 'Psychological and Emotional Impact of an HIV Diagnosis', *Nursing Times*, Vol 91. No 8, pp 37–39.

HOWARD, R (1995) 'Reasons for Older People Attending A&E', *Nursing Times*, Vol 91, No 13, pp40-43.

NAIDOO, N and WILLS, J (1994) *Health Promotion – Foundations for Practice*, Bailliere Tindall.

OPPENHEIM, AN (1992) *Questionnaire Design, Interviewing and Attitude Measurement*, Pinter.

ROBERTSON, J and ROBERTSON, J (1967) *Young Children in Brief Separation*, Tavistock Child Development Research Unit.

THORNES, R (1988) *Caring for Children in the Health Services – Hidden Children: An Analysis of ward attenders in children's wards*, HAWCH.

GLOSSARY

Analysis –

the process of interpreting **data**.

Bias –

any unintended influence on research that may distort the findings. For example, a researcher may inadvertently introduce bias by asking questions in a way that generates a response in favour of the researcher's view of a subject.

Central tendency –

a term used in statistics to describe the scores that can be identified as 'central' in the distribution of a set of figures. These measures include the **mean, median** and **mode**.

CD-ROM –

compact disc, read only memory; an abbreviation commonly used to describe computerised library indexes of published articles and books.

Closed question –

the kind of question in which a researcher expects a limited range of responses. For example, to the question 'Do you own a television set?' the respondents will be expected to answer 'yes' or 'no'. Contrasts with **open questions**.

Cluster sample –

a **sample** identified as a smaller group within the larger **population** being researched.

Content analysis –

the process of analysing **data** using words rather than figures.

Convenience sample –

a sample from a **population** selected on the basis of its accessibility to the researcher rather than on the basis of **random sample procedures**.

Data –

the information collected in the course of a research study. This may be in numerical form (**quantitative**) or in written or verbal form (**qualitative**).

Data collection techniques –

ways in which data or information can be collected, such as **questionnaires, interviews, observation** etc.

Deductive reasoning –

taking a known idea or theory and applying it to a situation (see also **inductive reasoning**).

Dependent variable (DV) –

the variable within a hypothesis which is affected by the **independent variable**.

Descriptive design –

an approach to research in which the researcher describes what is observed. There is no attempt to control or manipulate **variables** (in contrast to **experimental research** design).

Descriptive statistics –

a type of statistics used to describe and summarise **data**. For example, the data from a research study may be presented in percentages as a means of summarising large sets of data (see also **inferential statistics**).

Experimental design –

an approach to research in which the researcher controls the **independent variable** and measures the effect on the **dependent variable** in an attempt to look for a cause and effect.

Evaluation research –

a research method which attempts to establish the value of a programme. This may, for example, be a programme of study or a programme of health care. The value is determined by whether or not the programme achieves its goals or meets the needs of the users of the programme.

Event sampling –

an approach used in **observation** techniques of data collection in which the researcher begins the observation as the event occurs and continue until the event is completed. For example, a researcher studying a social worker's interactions with clients would begin the observation as the meeting between the social worker and the client begins and finish the observation as the meeting ends. Contrasts with **time sampling**.

Generalisability –

the extent to which the findings from a study **sample** can be generalised to the **population** from which the sample was taken.

Hypothesis –

a statement of a relationship between two or more **variables**. The hypothesis will always include at least one **independent variable (IV)** and at least one **dependent variable (DV)**. For example, 'eating excess calories (IV) will result in an increase of weight (DV)' (see also **null hypothesis**).

Independent variable (IV) –

the **variable** within a **hypothesis** which can be manipulated by the researcher. The independent variable will cause an effect on the **dependent variable**. For example, 'running (IV) will increase the heart rate (DV)'. In this case the researcher can manipulate the IV 'running' by controlling how much of this the subjects do.

Inductive reasoning –

using **observations** to formulate an idea or theory rather than taking known ideas or theories.

Inferential statistics –

a procedure in which statistical tests are used to infer whether the **observations** in the **sample** studied are likely to occur in a larger **population**.

Interview –

an approach used in research in which the researcher collects **data** by face-to-face contact with the subject being studied. One can use structured or semi-structured **questionnaires** in this approach.

Literature review –

a critical review of the literature relating to an area of research.

Literature search –

the process of finding published literature relating to an area of research.

Mean –

A measure used in **descriptive statistics** to identify the average score in a set of figures. It provides a means of summarising data and gives an indication of the **central tendency** of a set of figures.

Median –

a measure used in **descriptive statistics** to indicate **central tendency** in a set of figures by identifying the score which falls exactly in the middle of a set of figures.

Mode –

a measure used in **descriptive statistics** to describe the most frequently occurring number in a set of figures. This is a measure of **central tendency**.

Null hypothesis –

a hypothesis written in such a way as to indicate that there is no relationship between the **independent variable** and the **dependent variable**. For example, 'there is no relationship between running (IV) and heart rate (DV)'. Required for statistical testing procedures (see also **hypothesis**).

Observation –

a research method in which a researcher observes subjects in order to gather data. Observation research comprises both 'participation' and 'non-participation' research methods. The participant observer observes the subjects from within by becoming a member of the group he or she is researching. The non-participant observer observes the subjects from without by observing the group as a researcher.

Open question –

a way of phrasing a question to gather **data** from respondents in a research study. The response requires the respondent to make an individual response. For example, the researcher may ask 'Please tell me what you think about...'. Contrasts with **closed question**.

Pilot study –

a test of a **research design** on a smaller scale than the main study. Allows a researcher to test whether a research design will actually work.

Population –

indicates the entire set of subjects in a given group that could form the focus of a study. For example, all people who own television sets could be a population (see **sample**).

Purposive sample –

a sampling technique used in qualitative research in which the researcher chooses the **sample** on the basis of known characteristics or experiences. For example, a study designed to find out how health visitors feel about working in inner-city locations would only involve health visitors who had that particular experience.

Qualitative research methods –

research methods which collect **data** concerning feelings. Open-ended questionnaires, interviews, video recordings and observations can all be used to collect and analyse non-numerical data. Contrasts with **quantitative research methods**.

Quantitative research methods –

research methods which collect **data** that can be summarised numerically. Questionnaire scales, attitude scales, personality tests, physiological measurements and score sheets are all examples of this type of research method.

Questionnaire –

a tool for data collection in research. May be highly structured and contain only **closed questions** or have low structure and contain many **open questions**. It is not unusual for questionnaires to have a mix of both open and closed questions.

Quota sample –

a sampling technique designed to collect **samples** from a number of selected groups, e.g. a group of physiotherapists, a group of social workers or a group of nurses.

Random sample –

an approach to selecting a **sample** which ensures each member of the **population** being studied has an equal chance of being selected.

Range –

a measure used in **descriptive statistics** to indicate the difference between the highest and lowest scores in a set of figures.

Reliability –

the ability of a measurement procedure to produce the same results when used in different places by different researchers. An example of this could be a tape measure as this reliably measures length regardless of when, where or by whom it is used.

Research design –

refers to the overall plan for **data** collection and **analysis** in a research study.

Research process –

used to describe the actual procedures involved when implementing a **research design**.

Research question –

the question set at the beginning of a research project which may be developed to test the stated aims or a **hypothesis** (can also be referred to as the research problem).

Sample –

a subset of a particular **population** being studied. There are several different approaches to sampling (see **cluster, convenience, purposive, quota, random** and **stratified samples**).

Standard deviation (SD) –

a measure used in **descriptive statistics** to measure the degree of variability of a set of scores. The sum resulting from the statistical test used to calculate the SD indicates how much a set of figures is dispersed from the mean score.

Stratified sample –

a technique in which **random sampling** can be used to select people from two or more strata of the **population** independently. For example, a researcher completing a study of midwives could incorporate the views of junior and senior midwives by selecting a random sample from each of the two groups, rather than selecting a random sample from an overall population of midwives.

Structured questionnaire –

the type of **questionnaire** which consists of **closed questions** which give it a high level of structure (contrasts with semi-structured questionnaires which may contain more **open questions**).

Time sampling –

an approach to **observation** research in which the researcher undertakes observation in blocks of time. For example, a researcher may be observing how care is organised in a hospital ward over a 24-hour period in short blocks of 2 hours' observation. Contrasts with **event sampling** in which the researcher may only observe a specified event.

Triangulation –

the use of more than one method of collecting or interpreting **data**. For example, using **observation** and **interviews** or structured **questionnaires** and interviews.

Validity –

the extent to which a research tool measures what it is supposed to measure.

Variable –

the term used to describe the characteristics or features of the objects or people in a research study. For example, variables that may be studied in relation to people are hair colour, weight, height, etc., whilst 'objects' studied could include a wound dressing, a teaching programme, a dietary regime, etc. (See also **independent variable** and **dependent variable**.)